The Weeping Willow

The Weeping Willow

Encounters with Grief

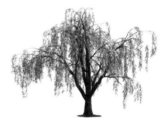

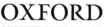

Lynne Dale Halamish
and Doron Hermoni

OXFORD
UNIVERSITY PRESS
2007

OXFORD
UNIVERSITY PRESS

Oxford University Press, Inc., publishes works that further
Oxford University's objective of excellence
in research, scholarship, and education.

Oxford   New York
Auckland   Cape Town   Dar es Salaam   Hong Kong   Karachi
Kuala Lumpur   Madrid   Melbourne   Mexico City   Nairobi
New Delhi   Shanghai   Taipei   Toronto

With offices in

Argentina   Austria   Brazil   Chile   Czech Republic   France   Greece
Guatemala   Hungary   Italy   Japan   Poland   Portugal   Singapore
South Korea   Switzerland   Thailand   Turkey   Ukraine   Vietnam

Published by Oxford University Press, Inc.
198 Madison Avenue, New York, New York 10016

www.oup.com

Oxford is a registered trademark of Oxford University Press

Library of Congress Cataloging-in-Publication Data
Halamish, Lynne Dale.
The weeping willow : encounters with grief /
by Lynne Dale Halamish and Doron Hermoni.
p. cm.
ISBN: 978-0-19-532537-9 (pbk.)
1. Grief.   2. Bereavement—Psychological aspects.   3. Death—Psychological aspects.
I. Hermoni, Doron.   II. Title.
BF575.G7H337 2007
155.9'37—dc22   2006038892

1 3 5 7 9 8 6 4 2

Printed in the United States of America
on acid-free paper

For El Roei

Foreword

⌒

Truth and Honesty

People living their life and coming to its end are there for all of us to see. We think we know about life and how to live it, how to love and how to be bereft, because these things are ubiquitous and right before our eyes. Those who take care of others— for example, counselors, psychologists, nurses, and physicians— are especially privileged to be a part of the lives of others and to have the opportunity to gain understanding of sickness, suffering, and troubles.

The fact is, however, that most people do not learn from others, and even those who by profession should know the most about life and death or love and grief often seem lacking in this regard. Why do people see but not see, listen but not hear? Goethe said that one sees what one knows, or, turned around, what you already know tells you what you are seeing and tells you what the words you are hearing mean. There is a kind of puzzle that asks you what is missing from a picture. People consistently fail the test. They see what they expect to see even when it is not there. Conversely, they do not see what is there if they do not expect it. All this is a complicated way of saying that perception—for example, sight, hearing, or touch—is thinking, not just sensing. This implies that misconceptions lead to misperceptions. We are filled way above our earlobes with misconceptions about people, life, love, loss, and grief. Think, for example, about the many different psychological theories you have heard which purport to explain human behavior, or even the different ideas you have personally about why people do what they do. If you are explaining the same thing a dozen different ways, it means you do not understand it.

Grief is particularly troublesome to know about and to deal with. Death is surrounded by emotional pain, before, during, and for a long time afterward. People often react to the emotional distress of others by dread, denial, or learned stereotypes. Sadly, professionals also have these same reactions. Afraid to see pain, they see what they know; afraid to hear, they do not listen. They may not know what to say or how to behave—who would teach them? In parts of the contemporary world, murder, war, and terrorism have produced death beyond comprehension. Drowning in grief, people still have difficulty knowing what to do. Teaching about grief is, by the nature of the subject, problematic.

All of which is why this is such a remarkable book. What is it? Short stories about people who are dying or who are grieving (or both), followed by a few distilled truths about people and responses to grief emerging from the story, followed by quotations from the academic literature. Simple enough; so why is it exceptional? Because the stories are filled with unadorned truths about people living through life's hardest moments. Lynne Halamish and Doron Hermoni can see what is there, see through the emotion to the people living it. Even more than seeing, they can hear what is said. These authors can do what most of us cannot: uncover the truth in the midst of human suffering. Then, equally unusual, they can reveal it to us in few words. As in Käthe Kollwitz's famous sketch *The Call of Death*—not a wasted line.

In addition to telling the truth, and despite how succinct they are, the stories are real. I do not believe you will have any difficulty knowing that these are actual people and their suffering is real. (Your tears will also confirm this.) So is their humor.

The authors did not write this book just to tell stories; they are teachers, and their narratives are meant to teach. To teach the grieving that what is happening to them and what they feel has been experienced by others, to teach those who must live and deal with the grief of others how best to act and what to say (or not say), and to teach professionals how to work with those in their care who are dying or grieving. That pretty much covers all of us, doesn't it? In fact, this is a book about persons with a universal trouble—loss comes to all.

Earlier, I said that all perceptions are colored by thought and beliefs. These authors seem to be able to see what is actually there—the thing itself. A psychologist once wrote, "Data without theory are like babies without parents: their life expectancy is low." What is Halamish and Hermoni's theory? Their theory is *no theory*. Learn to see what actually is, to hear every word, see every expression, and attend to everything that makes up the context, and these will tell you the truth of the thing. The stories speak for themselves; no theory is needed. What sets this work apart is the authors' inherent honesty—their rare ability to see and hear what is, let their perceptions take them where they go, no matter how painful, and then find the words to express them simply and teach us. Remarkable.

Eric J. Cassell, MD
Clinical Professor of Public Health, Weill Medical College
    of Cornell University
Attending Physician to Inpatients,
    New York–Presbyterian Hospital
Minisink Hills, Pennsylvania
2007

Preface

‿

THE WEEPING WILLOW is a collection of true stories about death, dying, and grieving, stories based on field experiences and on knowledge from many other sources.

The target audience includes the comforter as well as the griever—not necessarily the professional, although every professional who lives long enough will eventually become the griever.

The distinguishing features of this book are its brevity and its directness. The model is laser surgery; each story focuses on very few points, preferring clarity to mass. The goal is to provide practical tools for the griever and/or the comforter or professional.

If there is no practical approach to the specific dilemma, you will not find a story about it in this book.

The book works on three levels: (1) clinical stories; (2) brief theoretical background; and (3) tools at a glance. Our premise is that theory is not enough, tools are not enough, and stories are not enough, but together they can flesh each other out and make useful instruments for the reader. Each story or chapter in the book contains a vignette along with the teaching that can be gleaned from it. The stories are brief, one to three pages long, and so is the teaching. The work is designed to be a handbook, offering guidelines to assist the reader in times of personal grief or the grief of those near him or her both personally and professionally. Each teaching contains two to four tools for dealing with death.

Many types of grief are addressed between its covers, from the lingering bleakness of slow gradual death, to the disorienting trauma of sudden unexpected death; from death by natural causes to death by suicide or terrorist bombing; from the death of a spouse, grandparents, or parents to the death of children or siblings.

The Weeping Willow is not meant to replace counseling; rather, it is an addition to the arsenal of counseling. It is also, on some level, a "call to order" to counselors, other professionals, and friends who have not been trained for grief counseling and are using impractical or erroneous methods.

This book is also meant to provide some assistance to those who would not otherwise get counseling or where grief counseling is unavailable or unnecessary. It is meant to normalize normal grief responses—to reassure the grievers and those around them that they are not "crazy" for experiencing a less understood but valid aspect of grief.

The tools you will find here are not the only ones—there are other effective tools in the field of grief counseling—but these are gleaned from the field, have been tested there, and work well. However, our advice to the reader is the advice we also use: "If it works for you, use it. If it doesn't, throw it away." No reservations, no sentiment; be practical.

Do not lose yourself in the field, whether that field is your profession or your family and friends. Every meeting between two people is two worlds colliding, sometimes roughly, and sometimes with a gentle nudge. Although you may use the tools in this book, do not ignore yourself when you do so. Be present as who you are. A tool needs to be appropriate to the person using it, or at least to part of the personality. Take chances. There will never be enough tools for dealing with death.

We leave you with the blessing of Jonathan Swift: "Live every day of your life."

Acknowledgments

WE WOULD LIKE TO EXPRESS heartfelt thanks to:

All of the people who generously allowed us to use their stories to teach others to recover from loss, without whom there certainly would be no book.

Eric Cassell, an amazing, brilliant man who has become a dear friend. Eric made us believe, throughout the project, that this book could be and needed to be written. Eric walked us through each chapter, and his presence can be felt throughout the book.

Hannah Weiss, generous friend and wise woman, for invaluable accurate and pointed feedback and initial editing.

Lisa Loden, dear friend, for kind assistance with proofreading and support all the way through.

Sissy Soref, for valuable, insightful research.

Peter Rowan and Al Evers, for generous permission for use of the lyrics of "Waiting for Elijah."

Maya Karmi-Dror, for great assistance with the cover photo.

Oxford University Press, especially Shelley Reinhardt, Abby Gross, and Christi Stanforth, for their warm interest and guidance.

Doron would also like to thank:

Miki, my wife, friend, and partner, who taught me the power of life and hope. For her support and inspiration, with love.

To my future—Oded, Saar, Omri, and Netta—for bringing joy and love to my life.

My parents and extended family, who taught me so much on life and death.

My coauthor, Lynne, for her vision and courage to accomplish a dream.

Lynne would also like to thank:

Asaf, husband, life partner, and best friend for moment-by-moment support, clarity, vision, and encouragement through life, work, and the book.

Shachar, Hilah, and Oriah, my kids and my joy, for listening, giving support, ideas, love, and clear feedback all the way through.

Zohar, my stepson, who taught me more about love and loss than any other person.

Toni, Jordan, Rachel, and Naomi, my siblings, for support and encouragement.

Rachel-Rachel, Marianna, Adidush, and Francie, for active assistance and encouragement.

Rachelli Hacham, my sister-in-law, for the right word at the exact right moment.

Doron, my coauthor, for being a partner in this vision.

And, of course, primarily, the one true G-d, creator of heaven and earth, without whom we cannot breathe or function and are hopelessly lost.

Contents

$\backsim$

Grief Map

⌒

This is a "Road Map of Grief." It is designed to help you find your way around if you don't want to read the entire book and are looking only for practical tools to deal with a specific situation.

HOW TO USE THE MAP

1. In the top row, find the relationship that is the subject of your concern.

2. In the left-hand column, find the specific issue that concerns you.

3. The intersection of these two items will direct you to the relevant chapter(s).

Grief Map

ISSUE OF CONCERN	RELATIONSHIP						
	CHILDREN	TEENAGERS	SIBLINGS	PARENTS	WIDOW(ER)/PARTNER	DYING PERSON/SERIOUSLY ILL PERSON	ADULTS
Truth telling	2, 8	3, 11	30	6, 9, 14		4, 6, 12, 18	17, 24, 27, 28
Practical solutions	1, 8, 21	3, 15	25, 30	6, 9, 14, 16, 19, 22	13, 24	4, 6, 7, 12, 18	5, 17, 20, 24, 25, 27
Perception and language	1, 2, 10, 21	11, 15	30	9, 23	13, 23, 24	4, 7, 12, 18	17, 20, 24, 26, 27, 28
Listening	1, 2, 8, 10, 21	3, 11, 15		1, 6, 9, 16, 23	23	4, 6, 7, 12, 18	17, 26
Cost vs. benefit	23			6, 14, 16, 19, 22	13, 24	4	24
Talking about death	1, 2, 8, 10, 21	3, 11, 15	5, 25, 30	6, 9, 14, 16, 22, 29	13, 24	4, 6, 12, 18	5, 20, 24, 25, 26, 27, 28
Preparation for death	2			6, 14, 16, 22	24	4, 6	17, 24, 28
Decision making	8	3, 15	25, 30	6, 9, 14, 19	13, 24	6, 7, 12	17, 24, 25
Saying goodbye	2		5	6, 14, 22	24	4, 6, 18	5, 24
Hope/meaning	8	3, 11		9, 19	24	7	24

ISSUE OF CONCERN	CHILDREN	TEENAGERS	SIBLINGS	PARENTS	WIDOW(ER)/ PARTNER	DYING PERSON/ SERIOUSLY ILL PERSON	ADULTS
Timing of death	2			6, 22		6	
Lingering death	2			6, 14, 19, 22		4, 6, 12, 18	17, 24
Sudden death	1, 8	3, 11, 15	30	9, 23	23		
Funeral	10			9, 24	24		24
Grief rituals			5, 25	14			6, 25, 26
Repercussions of loss	8, 10, 21	3, 11, 15	5, 25, 30	9, 19, 22, 23, 29	13, 23		17, 20, 25, 26, 27
Length of grief	8	11					
Returning to life after loss	21	3	30	9, 29	13	7	5, 20
Transference	1, 8	15				12	1, 20, 27
Body language	1, 21			9		4, 7, 18	20
Suicidal intent		15			15		17

The Weeping Willow

.

You Don't Know Till You Ask

⌒

JUMPING TO CONCLUSIONS, SPEAKING TO CHILDREN

TALKING TO CHILDREN about death is not considered easy. So when I assigned this task to students in the class on grief and mourning in the medical school, I decided to interview a child about death in front of the class.

I walked into the class and told them, "Today, we will have a guest lecturer, Boaz, age seven, whom I will interview with three questions about death." Their response, even to the prospect of witnessing this interview, was panic:

"What if he starts crying?"

"He won't start crying."

"But what if he does?"

"Okay, go get some tissue."

"Does his mother know he's coming?"

"Well, she didn't agree to give him the car today, so we had to tell her. What do you think? She is coming with him, of course."

Boaz had been asked to come and help me teach the students. He had also been informed that I would be asking him three questions about death. He did not know what the questions were in advance.

Boaz lost his father at the age of three. His only request prior to the class interview was that I not ask him to speak about his father, and I agreed.

Boaz and his mother enter the room. I call Boaz up to the front and introduce him: "Our guest lecturer today is Boaz. Boaz, could you come here please?" Boaz comes forward to me. "Boaz is seven years old. He will be our guest lecturer today. Boaz has come to help us understand more about kids so we can be better doctors."

To Boaz: "Could you please sit on the desk?" He clambers up on the desk, sits, and I sit beside him in a chair. His eye level is higher than mine intentionally. This is to give him a feeling of control in a daunting situation. *To the students*: "Pay attention to the vertical body language here."

"Boaz, you know I asked you to come here to talk to these students and help them learn about children and how they feel about death. Okay?"

"Yes."

"So I would like to ask you three questions."

"Okay."

"Are you ready?"

"Yes."

"Boaz, what is death?"

He is quiet and thoughtful, looking down and then to the side. Then he begins to speak in a slow, thoughtful way. "Death, um, is kind of like fainting, only you don't wake up. The heart stops beating, the breathing stops. Like fainting only you don't wake up. Death is really, really empty of life."

"That is a very good answer. Thank you."

"Boaz, what makes people die? What do people die from?"

Boaz speaks slowly and thoughtfully. "They fall off cliffs, they die in war, from a heart attack . . ." Silence.

"Does anything else make people die?"

"Yes, but I can't think of what right now." Acting light-hearted, rocking back and forth, he says, "Maybe terror bombings or stuff."

"Okay. Good work. Boaz, where are the dead?"

"The body or the soul?"

(Surprised.) "You pick."

"I know the body is in the grave."

"And the soul?"

"The good ones go to heaven. The bad ones go to hell."

"Where do the medium ones go?"

"Hmm, I don't know."

"Okay."

"Boaz, if any of the students here have questions for you, can they ask you?"

"No."

"Okay, thank you very much. You did a great job."

(The class applauds.)

Boaz and his mom leave to get something to drink in the cafeteria till class is over. I ask the class: "Was anyone surprised by the interview with Boaz?" The class gives a resounding affirmative.

"What surprised you?"

"He knew so much."

"He was so relaxed talking about death!"

"You could see his answers had a lot of thought behind them."

"He wasn't hurt or upset by the subject."

"What did you think about his answer to 'What is death'?"

"It was a great answer!"

"I really didn't know kids were so smart."

"What did you think of his answer about what causes death?"

"You could see he watches a lot of cartoons." All of the students laugh; I smile.

"Yeah, the falling off cliffs—ha ha!"

"Or maybe from action movies or computer games. Ha ha!"

I am still smiling. "That is a very interesting way to look at it." There is general laughter and an easy feeling in the class.

"How many of you watch cartoons or have ever watched them?" Everyone raises their hands.

"You weren't paying attention to the cartoons. When people fall off cliffs in cartoons, they don't die; they just get up again." The room is filled with a curious silence. "Boaz's father died in a sporting accident. He fell off a cliff." I see shock on a few faces, the color draining away.

Jumping to conclusions is dangerous and frequently incorrect. Almost always, the first answer to "What causes death?" that a child gives is related to the child's experience of the death of the person closest to him.

In the interview, when Boaz was asked "What causes death?" he answered in two ways, verbally and with body language. The first part of his answer was thoughtful and serious. When people talk about things that really matter to them, they are concentrated and focused. The second part of his answer, "Maybe terror bombings or stuff," he said in a very lighthearted way, rocking back and forth, despite the impact of his words on others.

When people talk about things that don't matter to them, that haven't affected them personally, they more frequently speak in a casual or lighthearted manner. I couldn't ask Boaz in the class why he said people die from falling off cliffs. Why? Because I asked his permission for an interview of three questions about death. He agreed on condition that he wouldn't be asked about his father's death. This was our contract. I could not pursue his answers in a way that would break this contract.

Logically, we know that in cartoons people or characters don't die. Therefore, he couldn't have gotten that answer from television. During the feedback session with the students, it was clear where they were going with the cartoon assumption. I gave them a lot of rope before I told them how Boaz's father had died. This was to bring the point home so they would learn that you don't know until you ask. People see what they want to see, hear what they want to hear. This does not serve the child. We need to see what is there, to see the person in front of us.

Pay attention to both body and verbal language. Put aside preconceptions as much as possible. Jumping to conclusions is a dangerous practice in child rearing, in medicine, and in counseling. It prevents us from connecting or communicating on a real level with the child.

"If you don't ask, you don't know." Over the years, I have met many people who tell me they can "feel" the person they speak to. They "just know" what the person is going through. This is a real thing. You may have a feeling. Your feeling may be correct. But you have one piece of information, and until you support it with a fact, by asking and confirming that feeling, you can't be sure. Remember, fact is fact and interpretation is interpretation. You have to know what you know and you have to know what you think, and most important, you have to know the difference between them.

To act on your feelings without first ascertaining the facts has three disadvantages with children. (1) You aren't allowing them to express themselves and to say something that's important to them. (2) You will not find out what they believe to be true or be able to help them to deal with damaging misconceptions about death. (3) You are not able to see their "truth" without their help because your own "truth" gets in the way.

The three questions I asked Boaz—What is death? What causes death? and Where are the dead?—are three basic questions about death that are frequently asked by children and more frequently concern them. This interview was designed to help break the taboo of speaking about death and specifically to help break the taboo of speaking to children about death. Breaking this taboo is very important if children are to receive their rightful place in the family in times of a family member's serious illness or death. When children do not receive this place in the family as mourners, they suffer isolation at precisely the time when they most need support.

CONCLUSIONS

- *If you do not ask, you do not know.*
- *Talk to children. They know more than you think.*
- *Pay attention to the way a child gives an answer both verbally and affectively (through his body language).*

REFERENCES

1. "Valuing children of all ages and respecting their views is more likely to encourage the development of successful relationships between you and your young patient" (Jonathan Silverman, Suzanne M. Kurtz, & Juliet Draper, *Skills for Communicating with Patients*, 2nd ed. [Abingdon: Radcliffe Publishing Ltd., 2005], p. 224).

2. "Studies have shown that even young children have quite well developed concepts relating to death and are able, with help, to understand that death is permanent, universal, irreversible, has a cause, and involves separation, and that dead people are different from live people in a number of respects (for example, they cannot move, feel, or eat)" (R. Lansdown & G. Benjamin, "The Development of the Concept of Death in Children Aged 5–9 Years," *Child: Care, Health and Development* 1 [1985]: 13–20).

2

The Weeping Willow

⌒

CHILDREN DEALING WITH IMPENDING DEATH

THREE-YEAR-OLD SHACHAR went up to the bed in the bedroom where her grandmother was lying unconscious. Gramma had been deteriorating with cancer for the past year. In the past week, she had entered the home hospice program and had lost consciousness twenty-four hours prior to this meeting. Shachar picked up her grandmother's limp hand in her own small hands and started to tell her what she had done that day. "Gramma, today in the play group we learned how to make things from PlayDoh. It has a funny smell"—she wrinkled her little nose—"but I like the way it feels."

Shachar's mother, Dale, thought Shachar would pick up on what was going on, that her grandmother was dying, by seeing that Gramma was unconscious. In fact, Shachar did not recognize that, so Dale had to take a more direct approach to make the parting effective.

Dale squatted down and put her arm around Shachar's shoulder. Shachar looked up. "Shachar, Gramma doesn't want to be sick anymore. She doesn't want to hurt anymore." She paused. "Shachar, Gramma wants to die and go to be with G-d." Shachar turned to look at her grandmother lying unconscious and then back at her mother.

"Shachar, it's time to say goodbye to Gramma."

Shachar gently laid her grandmother's hand down on the covers and went to the head of the bed.

"Pick me up higher, Mom." And when raised to her grandmother's level, she put her hand on Gramma's shoulder and kissed her on the cheek. "Bye-bye, Gramma."

Dale was stunned. How could this child kiss that face? Be so unaffected by the half-open eyelids, the gaping toothless mouth? Dale put her down and then gave Gramma a kiss of her own on the forehead. "Bye, Mom. I love you," she said quietly. Then Dale led Shachar out of the room into the living room before returning to Gramma's side.

Dale returned to the room, and Gramma breathed her last. About thirty seconds had passed since Shachar left the room.

Six years later, when Shachar was nine, she was walking with her mother in a field when they saw a majestic weeping willow tree. "That was Gramma's favorite tree," Shachar said. "It really was," replied Dale with surprise. "What else do you remember about Gramma?" Shachar related many things that Dale knew she herself had intentionally planted as memories of Gramma for Shachar.

Then Shachar said, "And I remember the day Gramma died."

"What do you remember about that day?"

"I remember that someone woke me up and drove me to Gramma's house, and it was the middle of the night." She paused. "You took me into the room where Gramma was lying on the bed. I went to talk to Gramma, and then you told me that Gramma doesn't want to stay alive anymore. That she wants to die and be with G-d."

"And then what happened?" Dale asked with curiosity.

"I gave Gramma a kiss goodbye, and she gave me the most beautiful smile!"

Dale was startled. There had been no smile. Shachar's grandmother had lain in bed unconscious, without her dentures, her mouth sunken and partially open, eyes half closed, pale, unlovely. At the time, Dale could hardly believe Shachar would want to kiss that face, well beloved though it had been. She began to wonder if perhaps Shachar had seen more of the reality than she herself had. Dale thought perhaps she herself was limited because of her locking on to the physical appearance and the disease.

Shachar is now twenty-one. She has a wonderful attitude toward death. She is the first to help friends and family when death approaches.

Should a child be told about an impending death? There are not many redeeming qualities about long, lingering death. But there is one really positive thing about it—time. However, this time is a positive thing only if you use it. Otherwise, it is just a longer period of suffering.

Why is this time so significant? Time is needed to adjust to the idea of the loss, both for the dying and for the loved ones. Time allows the opportunity to say some or all of the things we are denied the chance to say when the death is sudden and un-expected. Children also need time to adjust to the idea of im-pending death, when there is the opportunity. They also want to say goodbye or "I love you" or other things.

What should a child be told? Children do not need to know details of the illness prior to the death unless they have specific questions. They do need to know the name of the disease. This reduces the size of the fear to include one type of disease rather than the more generic "Gramma is sick," which can include everything from the common cold to AIDS as a potential source of fear of death. The main point is the reality of parting from their loved one permanently. They should be encouraged and supported in making final contact with their loved one in a way that is comfortable. So if someone who is significant to the child is going to die in the near future, the child, like the adult, de-serves both the knowledge that the death is impending and the opportunity to say goodbye.

When should a child be told? If someone who is significant to the child is going to die in the near future, the child, like the adult, deserves to know that the death is coming and be pro-vided with enough time and opportunity to say goodbye. It is usually best if the dying person is conscious and cognizant of his or her surroundings (see chapter 6, "Give Me Permission to Die"). Sometimes, we have less time available, for example, when the notice of the dying is the unconsciousness; then we have to make do with what we have. We do know, however, according to research, that there is a possibility that an uncon-scious person hears. Because of this, relatives, including children, can say goodbye even though there is no clear response from the dying person. We can see in this story that it is frequently very effective for the griever to say goodbye, especially if he or she knows that the dying person may be able to hear him or her.

What kind of protection does a child need? When we feel the urge to protect children from encounters with a dying loved one, we need to reevaluate what we mean by protection. At some point soon, whether we want it or not, the child will no longer have the dying relative. The choice is for the dying person to suddenly disappear from the child's world, or for the child to have the chance to say goodbye, perhaps express love or appreciation. Which is more protective? If children experience the sudden disappearance of a loved one, they may conclude that others can disappear just as easily, undermining their sense of security.

The younger the child, the less biased and acculturated (culturally conditioned) their view of the world will be, including illness and death. To that extent, they may have a tendency to interpret differently or even overlook details that an older person would find repulsive or depressing, as Shachar did. It is important not to assume that our own discomfort is the child's discomfort unless we have supportive evidence. At the same time, it is important to be alert to signs of discomfort (or lack of understanding) on the part of the child and to talk with him or her about these. This can help protect the child from misunderstandings about the dying they are witnessing.

If the dying person is attached to various machinery, such as life support, this might frighten children. These unfamiliar things, along with their purpose in helping the dying person, can be explained before the children see them. This will help children to navigate the new situation with more confidence.

CONCLUSIONS

- *Children, like adults, should be a part of the dying process of their close relatives.*
- *An effective way to protect children from the negative impact of sudden death is to allow them to say goodbye when the death is not sudden.*
- *Because we cannot protect children from the existence of death, a good way to help them cope is to give them the tools to deal with it. These include having the opportunity to say goodbye to dying relatives in a comfortable way, with just enough knowledge to deal with any potentially disturbing elements in the surroundings.*

REFERENCES

1. "Primary prevention involves preparing the child for bereavement[,] . . . explaining and talking openly with children about their experience, encouraging children's involvement in shared mourning practices and resumption of normal activities, and providing early professional help if needed. . . . Counseling after bereavement is one of the few preventive interventions shown to promote mental health in adults, and . . . there is no reason to believe that it is any less effective in children. . . . Understanding about death is the first step on the way to recovering from bereavement and can be helped by being sensitively prepared by trusted adults for seeing and touching the dead body and encouragement to attend the funeral" (D. Black, "Childhood Bereavement," *British Medical Journal* 312 [1996]: 1496).

2. "Children are rarely prepared for the death of a parent or a sibling, and yet we know from studies of bereaved adults that mourning is aided by a foreknowledge of the imminence and inevitability of death. Children who are forewarned have lower levels of anxiety than those who are not, even within the same family" (D. Black, "Coping with Loss: Bereavement in Childhood," *British Medical Journal* 316 [1998]: 931–933).

3. "Research supports the positive adaptive value of keeping children informed about the parent's illness and preparing them for the death. It is also helpful to provide them with opportunities to ask questions and to express their feelings, including negative ones, without social constraints. The physician can create such opportunities by offering to meet with the parents and adolescents together or separately and by suggesting relevant pamphlets, booklets, and Web sites (suggested resources are listed on the *Journal of the American Medical Association* Web site: www .jama.com). Adolescents also benefit from opportunities to review their understanding of the situation with parents, physicians, and other experts. When family communication about a parent's illness is avoided or unrealistic, the child's chances for a favorable outcome are compromised" (G. H. Christ, K. Siegel, & A. E. Christ, "Adolescent Grief—'It Never Really Hit Me . . . Until It Actually Happened,'" *Journal of the American Medical Association* 288 [2002]: 1269–1278).

3

Who Will Go to Torah with Me?

⌒

SECURITY FOLLOWING PARENTAL DEATH

JORDAN WAS TWELVE YEARS OLD, a religious Jewish boy sitting with his mother and four siblings in a neighbor's apartment, three days after his father's sudden death in a car accident. He was the youngest of five children. I had met the family only moments before during the formal seven-day mourning period known as "sitting Shiva." This family would have a difficult period of mourning because Jordan's mother, Karen, was receiving chemotherapy for advanced cancer. Joseph, Jordan's father, had been the anchor in the family since the onset of Karen's cancer five years previously. Now, in the wake of Joseph's death, the family was adrift on a wave of grief and insecurity.

I had called them out of their home, leaving behind those who came to comfort them. We were sitting in the neighbor's apartment. They all looked battered and bewildered by their grief and loss. There was only one place to start.

I addressed the new widow and slowly asked her questions about the death, giving time for her to answer all of the questions. "Karen, tell me what happened to your husband. How did you find out? Who told you? Do you remember the words they used? What did you do then? What were your first thoughts?"

It would be months before they realized the impact of this death. "Karen, what is the most difficult thing about your husband's death today?" She blurted out, "He never even said goodbye!" and burst into bitter tears, along with all the children. Gradually, the tears subsided. "He left me alone!" she wailed, and all the grief and pain burst forth anew.

After many tears, pauses, and new statements resulting in more tears, Karen had finally finished. I turned to the eldest child with the same question: "Moshe, what is the hardest thing about your father's death for you right now?" And he began his narrative of pain, one sentence at a time, each sentence followed by a fresh wave of grief, until he had no more to say. Then on to the next child. In order of age, we went around the room, a grueling, gut-wrenching experience for all.

We had been sitting for over two hours when Jordan's turn came. "And Jordan, what is the hardest thing about your father's death for you?"

Jordan looked at me with a forlorn expression. "Who will accompany me in my reading of the Torah?" Everyone burst into tears. Jordan's bar mitzvah, the milestone ceremony that marks the coming of age for a Jewish boy, was only a month and a half away. Like all fathers, his father was supposed to accompany him as he was called up in the synagogue to publicly read from the Torah scroll for the first time.

More tough questions followed. "Who will teach me to be a handyman?" (This was his father's profession.) "Who will help me with my homework?" Everyone was crying; comments like "Poor Jordan!" were interspersed with the sobs.

After a few minutes, the crying died down and the room became quiet. I looked at Jordan and asked, "Who will actually go with you to the Torah, Jordan?" A shocked silence followed. Jordan looked at me, and then his eyes wandered up and to the right. A few moments later, he focused once again on me and said, "Maybe my second brother, Josh?"

"He is sitting here. Ask him."

"Josh, would you stand up with me at my bar mitzvah?"

"Of course, of course!" Josh exclaimed, crying with the rest of the family.

"And, Jordan, who will teach you to be a handyman?"

"Maybe my big brother, Moshe?"

"He is sitting with us. Ask him."

"Moshe, would you teach me to be a handyman?"

"Yes, yes, my brother," Moshe replied emotionally and came over to hug Jordan.

"Jordan, who will help you with your homework?"

"Maybe my sister, Hannah?"

"She is sitting here. Ask her."

"Hannah . . ."

"You know I will, Jordy. I love you," Hannah interrupted.

The family meeting began with a "debriefing." The purpose of the debriefing is to place on the table for the whole family all of the information about the death that is available. This is partly so that no one feels left out and overlooked, and it also serves to reinforce normal grief responses and encourages the bereaved to say all of the things that they are feeling. This is where the normalcy of their responses can be confirmed (unless the responses turn out not to be normal). The debriefing also reconfirms the fact of the death itself, which in the case of sudden, unexpected death is a hard concept to digest.

What was the purpose of the questions that I gave back to Jordan? Was it to help Jordan finish with the grief by asking him to answer his own questions and fears? No. In fact, the opposite. Jordan had a survival fear that needed to be addressed first before he could be free to begin his grief. This is similar to a situation where two soldiers are together on the battlefield and one is killed. The surviving soldier can't take the time to grieve—he needs to keep shooting, or else he may also be killed. He will have to wait till he is safer before he can begin to grieve.

With children, the burning question after the loss of a parent is "Who will take care of me?" Jordan addressed this same question in a very practical way. In the religious life of a Jewish boy, the bar mitzvah is his rite of passage into adulthood at age thirteen. In a vivid way, it is a symbol of his survival.

Too often when dealing with children, we are tempted to give false reassurance with meaningless words—"It will be okay," "Time heals," and so on—instead of dealing with legitimate, practical concerns engendered by the tragedy. Asking Jordan to voice his own burning questions and then giving him the authority to make significant decisions in his life brings personal power into a powerless situation. It honors his decision-making capability, and it serves as a positive model for the rest of the family to deal constructively with his questions instead of sidestepping them.

CONCLUSIONS

- *After a family or group trauma, it is helpful to go over all of the details together in order to clarify what happened, normalize grief reactions, and avoid the isolation of any member.*
- *It is important to deal with survival fears prior to dealing with grief, especially with children under the age of sixteen.*
- *Every one of the survivors' questions is legitimate and deserves confirmation, as well as a chance to seek out an answer. This restores some measure of personal power to a grieving person, whether adult or child.*

REFERENCES

1. "Bereaved children have fears of abandonment, fear of the death of those they love and themselves, guilt and fear of retribution for imagined or actual transgressions, difficulties in attaching to new caretakers, and difficulties at school. These problems need specific work done by those who can communicate at the child's level, who understand children's thinking and can use play materials appropriate to the child's developmental level" (D. Black, "Coping with Loss: Bereavement in Childhood," *British Medical Journal* 316 [1998]: 931–933).

2. "We need to educate adults on children's need to make sense of events, by creating or constructing a narrative or total picture of what happened, even when children are quite small. . . . This is recommendable to prevent the event from having unnecessary consequences. If parents and children or adolescents experienced

the disaster together . . . detailed review should be done with all persons involved present, as this increases the chance of getting a full picture of what happened" (A. Dyregrov, "Family Recovery from Terror, Grief and Trauma," Center for Crisis Psychology, Bergen, Norway, e-mail: atle@uib.no, www.icisf.org, accessed January 26, 2007).

4

The Black Place

TALKING ABOUT FEARS

"TELL ME ABOUT your hospital stay last week."

"It was terrible." Yotam, a fifty-five-year-old man, followed with a detailed description: "I couldn't breathe. I felt I was choking. We had no alternative so again I went to be hospitalized so they could help me."

"How do you feel when you have a setback like this?"

"I can't talk about it."

"Can you speak to your wife about your feelings when something like this happens?"

"No, I go to my room and sleep and sit alone and cry. It's that 'Black Place,' and I can't talk to anyone about it."

A few moments of heavy silence fell in the room.

"Under what circumstances could you speak about the Black Place?"

"I don't understand your question."

"If you could speak about the Black Place, in what place would you be able to speak about it? In the hospital? At home? Someplace else?"

There was a pause.

"At home. Only at home. No place else."

"If you could talk about the Black Place, to whom would you be able to speak about it? To a doctor? To extended family? To your wife? To a professional?"

He paused. "Only to my wife. To no one else. To you or to my wife."

"You said you can't talk to your wife about it."

Yotam answered with a troubled expression on his face. "No, I can't talk to her about it."

"Could you talk with me about the Black Place?"

"Ummm, I think so."

"We are in your home, and I am here." I paused. "Can we talk about the Black Place?"

"I can't talk about the Black Place." There were a few moments of silence.

"Yotam, you know the counseling business; psychology, social work, counseling—it is a huge business."

Yotam nodded silently looking a bit confused by the change of direction.

"You know that this whole huge business is actually based on one concept, one thought, one sentence?"

He looked at me with a puzzled frown. "It is?"

"Yes. Do you want to know what that thought or concept is?"

"Okay."

"It is the concept that if you speak about your feelings, they lose some of their power. Fears that are spoken about become less frightening."

I paused. "I want to help you, Yotam. But I can't do it alone."

He considered this for a while and then said, "I'll be right back."

Yotam rose laboriously from his chair and went to the bathroom. He washed his face, brushed his teeth, combed his hair, washed his hands, and came back to sit down in his chair. He gripped the arms of the chair and said, "Okay."

"Yotam, we are going to do this with ground rules. At any point while we are talking, if you say stop, I will stop immediately. You have control over this conversation. Is that clear?"

"Yes." His grip on the arms of the chair did not relax.

"The Black Place, is it a place that is full, or is it a place that is empty?"

Yotam took some time to think. "Empty."

"The Black Place, is it a place of emptiness or a place of powerlessness?"

He again thought before answering. "Powerlessness."

"The Black Place, is it an existential fear?"

He paused to think. "Yes."

"Is existential fear essentially the fear of nonexistence?"

Yotam looked down, then raised his eyes to look at me. "Yes."

"What is another way to say nonexistence?"

"Emptiness."

"Is there another way to say it?"

"No."

"Is 'death' another way to say nonexistence?"

He looked down, then looked up with wet eyes. "Yes."

"Did you know, Yotam, that in a primitive culture some-where in Africa, they still worship stone idols? There is an idol, a stone statue that squats down with its elbows bent and palms up in the air like this." I demonstrated the position. "On the palms of this statue, there stands another, just like it, only eight or nine times bigger. The statue on the bottom is the idol of death. The much larger statue on the top is the idol of the fear of death. Do you think the proportions of these idols might be about right?"

Yotam looked startled and then replied, "Yes, I really think they are right."

"The fear of death can be a very scary thing. Everyone is afraid of death itself or of what death can take from them. Is fear of death the Black Place?"

Yotam nodded.

"What is the scariest thing about death for you?"

"What do you mean?"

"Is it the way or timing of death? Is it the uncertainty or lack of control? Is it nonexistence?"

"Lack of control . . . or nonexistence."

We continued to speak about the Black Place for the better part of an hour. Then we both sat in silence for a few minutes.

"Tell me, Yotam, look at the Black Place. How does it look now?"

He responded slowly, thoughtfully, and assuredly. "It is a little less black."

Talking about fears reduces them. Because Yotam couldn't speak about the Black Place with anyone, that, in effect, forced him to carry a heavy secret alone. Holding secrets tends to isolate the secret bearers. If they cannot speak of their great fears or concerns, these fears or concerns occupy their subconscious and conscious thoughts, taking their concentration and energy and making them tired or spacy. Holding important secrets requires a great deal of effort and comes with a price of lowered strength for other parts of life.

In the case of impending death, if both the support system and the dying person are pretending that everything is all right (a very common situation), then everyone is isolated by pretense, lies, or ignoring the situation. Speaking the word "death" does not summon death, but it does push isolation away. To talk about death, whether impending, as in Yotam's case, or death that has already taken place, requires two things: (1) someone to speak openly, to put the subject on the table, so to speak; (2) someone who is willing to listen without trying to avoid or change the subject. Because of the taboo surrounding death, neither of these is easy to find. It often seems an impossible task to talk openly about death, particularly to one who stands in its shadow. As it happens, it is not impossible. The first time is hard, but once the relief it brings is apparent, it becomes easier and easier each time.

CONCLUSIONS

- *Talking about fears usually reduces them.*
- *Keeping secrets isolates both the dying person and the support system.*
- *Keeping secrets requires physical, emotional, and mental energy.*
- *It is important to hear the person's language, their way of speaking, and respond to them in the same language.*

REFERENCES

1. "Fear of death is a common characteristic among palliative care patients. . . . The level of death fear, irrespective of age, decreased under the comprehensive care in a palliative setting. . . . Reducing death fear represents an important factor towards a good death. Hospice care is intended to decrease patients' death fear levels and to work towards the goal of a good death through comprehensive care, which includes physical, psychological, social, and spiritual cares" (J.-S. Tsai, C.-H. Wu, T.-Y. Chiu, W.-Y. Hu, & C.-Y. Chen, "Fear of Death and Good Death among the Young and Elderly with Terminal Cancers in Taiwan," *Journal of Pain and Symptom Management* 4 [April 29, 2005]: 344–351).

2. "Fearing death is a rational response. For too long, medicine has ignored this primeval fear. Increasingly, clinicians recognize and address end-of-life issues, facing patients' and our own emotional vulnerabilities in order to connect and explore problems and fears. Listening and learning from the patient guides us as we acknowledge much of the mystery that still surrounds the dying

process. Rarely is there a simple or right answer. An empathetic response to suffering patients is the best support. Support is vital in fostering the adjustment of patients. A silent presence may prove more helpful than well-meant counsel for many patients. . . . Empathy and taking the time to be present and listen to the patient are some of the most important aspects of caring for the dying patient and provide a fulfilling role for the team who share the journey" (R. T. Penson, R. A. Partridge, M. A. Shah, D. Giansiracusa, B. A. Chabner, & T. J. Lynch Jr., "Fear of Death," *Oncologist* 10 [2005]: 160–169).

3. "Confidentiality is an essential ethical standard in medical practice, but secrets are destructive to healthy family function-ing" (M. Karpel & E. Strauses, *Family Secrets, Family Evaluation* [New York: Gardener Press, 1983], quoted in S. H. McDaniel, T. L. Campbell, J. Hepworth, & A. Lorenz, *Family Oriented Primary Care* [New York: Springer, 2005], p. 405).

5

The Tree

∽

IT IS NORMAL TO GROW
AFTER TRAUMA

"COME WITH ME to the garden," I said to Sarah. She looked a bit startled but came with me uncertainly. We walked over to a large bush. "Look at this bush. I pruned it a while ago." She glanced at the bush and looked back at me blankly.

"What do you see?"

"A bush?"

"Look closer," I said as I parted a clump of leaves to expose the end of the branch I had pruned.

Sarah looked carefully. "I see leaves growing, very lush, very green."

"What else do you see?"

"Well, all of the leaves are growing out of the sides of the branch."

"What do you see at the end of the branch?"

"A stump of the branch. This is where you pruned it."

"Right. This is the point of trauma. The bush has been through a trauma. The trauma killed part of it. Nothing grows from the pruned end. It is dry and slightly shriveled." I paused. "No leaves grow from that spot, but from the sides of the branch, in every direction, is life, new growth, and health. After a trauma, even after a death, or many deaths, there is the possibility, even the natural desire to return to life, to connect and to grow. We usually cannot grow in the same way or direction we had originally grown. Perhaps the previous choices have become irrelevant, but growth happens nonetheless."

Sarah had grown up with many losses, the most poignant of which, in childhood, had been her mother's repeated declaration that she never wanted her but wanted a boy instead.

Sarah left her native South America, like so many others, to come to Israel. The distance from the family yoke that she had lived under was a welcome change. She raised a family and lived communally, with high ideals, on a kibbutz. When the kibbutz dissolved, it was just one more link in a chain of losses. Her father died; her siblings all died. She brought her aging mother to Israel so Sarah could look after her despite their difficult relationship. Nothing had changed; her mother's song was the same with a new twist: "If only you had died instead of your siblings." She came to me to work on her losses, many losses, deaths among them. There was a fear of great power within her, a fear of being erased.

"We are born with an empty backpack on our shoulders," I said to Sarah. "All of our lives we are picking up stones and rocks and putting them into the backpack. Some of them are very small, and others are large and heavy. The stones that we carry are often difficult experiences, frequently involving loss or trauma. How long do we carry them? Until we empty the backpack—if we ever do. If we don't empty it, the weight accumulates, getting heavier and heavier as we age. Some of the stones we can throw away, some we cannot throw away, but even with these permanent stones we can take each one out, one by one, work with it, cut it down, shrink its size and weight. This is something that grief can be likened to. We work with the weight, reducing it, refining it. If we choose not to work with it, then grief accumulates. Holding it back begins to require a great deal of strength. This strength to hold the grief back becomes unavailable for other life functions. We become tired and can invest less and less in life."

With Sarah, the refining took the shape of separation. There had been no opportunity for separation, no opportunity to say goodbye. This was not because all of the deaths were sudden; some of them were, but she had had no tools to work with to accomplish separation.

So Sarah began to write letters to her dead.

Sarah went home, waited till she was alone, turned off the phone, and locked the doors. She prepared a workplace with tissues, a jug of water and a glass, a block of paper and several pens. She sat down and chose to write to her brother. She had not been able to stop thinking about him for weeks. She began to write. "Dear Sergio, it has been two years since I learned of your death, and three since we last spoke. I have some things to tell you." She then wrote all of the things she had been unable to say because of time and physical and emotional distance. She went over all the things she wished had been different. She wrote about regrets, joys, her feelings for him, both good and bad. And finally, after half an hour of tearful writing, she wrote, "Goodbye, baby brother."

Initially, Sarah had been hesitant to try the exercise, but after she wrote the first letter, she felt relieved. She began to write letters to all her dead. She finished writing when she wrote her seventh letter.

After writing the letters, she came back to meet with me and decide what to do with them. She decided to find a tree, dig a hole, put the letters in the hole, and plant the tree on top of them. But how would she find the right tree? Which tree would be appropriate? She waited for the "perfect one."

Sarah finally found a huge old tree that had been cut off at ground level; all of its seven massive branches had been cut into short stubs, and it had been lying dead on the ground for several months. She had to get a tractor with a lift to move it. She also had to dig a giant, deep hole to accommodate it for deep planting because no roots remained to steady it.

She decided to use this experience for an art project and documented the whole process photographically. The photographs show the hole and the tree suspended in the lift above the hole while Sarah drops all the letters in. In one of the photographs, the letters are fluttering down into the darkness of the hole. Another shows the planting of the tree and packing it in with dirt to steady its massive bulk. Sarah then watered the ground around the dead tree to compact the soil and anchor the dead tree more solidly into the ground. She then had someone take pictures of her decorating the tree with various clay pots, heavy ropes, and many other things.

A few weeks later, Sarah came to see me. She was withdrawn and contemplative as she related to me that the dead tree had begun to sprout leaves! She later brought more photos, and, indeed, the dead tree was covered with leaves. It had no roots, it had lain outside the ground for a very long time, and yet it lived.

Sarah and I discussed the symbolic significance of this "return from death." What did it mean to be replanted in another country without roots or support and flourish nonetheless?

CONCLUSIONS

- *It is normal to grow and reconnect with life after trauma. But the direction of one's life frequently changes.*
- *When there is no opportunity for separation before a death, it is still possible to effect a separation after the death, for example, through a letter.*
- *If we don't examine and work through our losses, we must continue to think about them, worry about them, or deny them, all of which take emotional strength and get in the way of living our lives.*

REFERENCES

1. "Putting upsetting experiences into words, including disclosure about emotions in response to the death of a spouse, is associated with improved physical and mental health. Written and oral disclosure studies have even demonstrated a positive influence on immune function. Based on these findings, physicians

might encourage bereaved patients to express their thoughts and feelings about the loss (e.g., in a journal)" (H. G. Prigerson & S. C. Jacobs, "Caring for Bereaved Patients: 'All the Doctors Just Suddenly Go,'" *Journal of the American Medical Association* 286 [2001]: 1369–1376).

2. "Many people are exposed to loss or potentially traumatic events at some point in their lives, and yet they continue to have positive emotional experiences and show only minor and transient disruptions in their ability to function. Unfortunately ... loss and trauma theorists have often viewed this type of resilience as either rare or pathological. The author challenges these assumptions by reviewing evidence that resilience represents a distinct trajectory from the process of recovery, that resilience in the face of loss or potential trauma is more common than is often believed, and that there are multiple and sometimes unexpected pathways to resilience" (G. A. Bonanno, "Loss, Trauma, and Human Resilience: Have We Underestimated the Human Capacity to Thrive After Extremely Aversive Events?" *American Psychologist* 59 [2004]: 20–28).

3. "Work through to the pain of grief. Identify and express the feelings related to the loss. Be in touch with yourself and what you are feeling—sadness, relief, whatever. The hardest feelings to work through are anger, guilt, anxiety, and helplessness. The common way to avoid this task is not to feel. Bury the feelings. But as someone once said, when you bury feelings, you bury them alive. And they will find some other ways of expressing themselves" (J. W. Worden, *Grief Counseling and Grief Therapy: A Handbook for the Mental Health Practitioner* [New York: Springer, 1991]. Quoted in Jack Genskow, Ph.D., "Responding to Loss: A Practical Framework," at www.post-polio.org/ipn/pnn12–3.html #jack, accessed January 12, 2007).

6

Give Me Permission to Die

$\backsim$

TALKING OPENLY ABOUT DEATH

HER MOTHER SENT the nurse to call Rachel into the room. Rachel came and sat down near the bed in the comfortable, homey bedroom.

"Rachel, I don't want to live anymore. I am tired and hurting. I have had enough. I want to go be with G-d."

"Mom," answered Rachel, "I don't understand what you are asking me for." During Rachel's medical career, patients who were hopelessly ill, and even some who weren't, had asked her to end their lives, their suffering. Is that what her mother was asking her now? She knew she could not do it.

"I just want you to give me permission to die," her mother answered.

"Permission?" Rachel responded, disarmed. She thought about how she had come to be with her mother. She moved her family and profession from the East Coast to the West, settling in for the long haul when the diagnosis came a year earlier: colon cancer, metastasized.

She thought of the long years of study and living so far away for so long. She remembered the huge phone bills, missing her mother so much, hour-long audio tapes sent back and forth, videos of the kids. Then, finally, deciding to uproot yet again to give her children their grandmother. Her mother, Katherine, a wonderful, vibrant woman, was so dissimilar to the thin, tired woman lying in the bed before her. Rachel had had less than a year to enjoy her mother.

During the past year, since the diagnosis, they had talked daily, opening their hearts to each other. Rachel had asked her mother what she would've done differently if she could change the past, and what she would've kept the same. They spoke together of thoughts, fears, dreams, disappointments, successes and failures, values and goals. It was the closest they had ever been. There had been tears, laughter, silence, confessions. At one point, about three months earlier, Rachel had donned her professional persona and said, "Mom, if this disease continues in the way it is going, there will be a point where you will lose consciousness. What would you like me to do then? Resuscitate? Hospitalize? Put you on a breathing machine? Intubation? Pain killers? What?"

Katherine had answered, "I don't want anything except pain control. I don't want to leave home, I don't want the hospital, I don't want to extend my life artificially."

Rachel had seen to the DNR (do not resuscitate) disclaimer and had left instructions by Katherine's bed in case she was not present when her mother lost consciousness.

And now her mother was giving up sooner than Rachel had expected.

"Mom," she began, then swallowed and began again. "Mom, do what is best for you. I will miss you terribly, but I will manage." Her eyes were wet.

Katherine placed her frail hand in Rachel's. "Thank you. Can you ask dad to come in?" Rachel kissed her mother tenderly on the forehead and went to call her father.

Katherine put the same question to Isaiah, her husband. The answer was curt and angry: "I am fifteen years older than you! You are not going to die! I want you to get better, get out of that bed, and start taking care of me!" Katherine sighed.

Katherine spoke with each of her six children over the next few days, asking each for permission to die. There were many tearful partings, each in its own way. Ruth, the youngest, could only speak by phone because she was living far from home and was unable to fly due to her advanced pregnancy.

After each acquiescence, Katherine would ask Isaiah again, and again he would refuse. Finally, with mounting pressure from the children, he gave in and gave permission for Katherine to die. Within the hour of receiving that sought-after permission, Katherine lost consciousness, as if to run before her husband could take his permission back.

Two days later, Katherine died peacefully, surrounded by family in her home. There were no heroic attempts to prolong her life. Her dying was as she wished, as she requested.

Why listen to the dying person? One of the most difficult things about terminal illness is the isolation it brings precisely because no one wants to really listen to dying persons. We are afraid of what they might say, of not knowing how to respond. We are afraid to talk about death as if the talk itself can call or bring the death. We act as if we are afraid of tempting fate. In Hebrew, we say, "Don't open your mouth to the devil"; it means it is never safe to talk about tragedy or death. But the fact is that death comes whether or not we talk about it. Death comes both to those who talk about it and to those who don't. But avoidance of the topic of death and frequently even of the dying person himself or herself can become so extreme that the dying person may go through a "social death" prior to the physical death. They are avoided by friends, family, and even hospital personnel. In the hospital, personnel may care for the patients without looking into their eyes or relating to them on any significant level. This can happen even when people come to visit but refuse honest or real communication with the dying person, choosing instead to skirt the subject, frequently filling in with platitudes such as "It will be fine. Everything will work out." This isolation unnecessarily increases the emotional pain of the dying person, which is already considerable.

In working with dying people, you will find that contrary to popular belief, the dying are usually very relieved to find someone with whom they can speak openly.

How do you start a discussion about death? Usually the first time, like many other things, is the most difficult. It helps to lean forward in your seat, meeting the person's gaze directly and asking, "How are you doing?" with intent to hear the truth. This intent is clear enough for them to understand. At this point, one of two things will probably happen. Either they will break eye contact and say, "I am not ready to talk about it," in which case you might respond, "Let me know when you are. I am available to listen"; or they will begin to tell their story. During the story, interrupt only to ask for clarification, in a low, quiet voice. Be careful not to break the flow of their speech. During the telling of the story, their eyes will usually intermittently meet those of the listener. When the story is finished, wait for their eyes to return to yours.

Then perhaps, begin to ask other questions. Frequently, very practical ones are useful, such as: "If you could pick anyone at all to raise your children, in the event that you cannot, who would it be and why?" or "What is the most important thing for you to do right now?"

Who frames the discussion? Well, usually the patient does. They decide when it has gone long enough or far enough for this meeting. They may pick up the same thread again the next time you meet. On the other hand, they may find another direction after having mulled over the discussion for a while.

When do you discuss the possibilities of loss and death? It is wise to take into consideration that when serious illness is involved, the ill person generally thinks of death as a possibility. Some people dwell on it constantly, while others push the thought away or only inspect it as a stray thought now and again. It is good to have the discussion early, when the affected person is still energetic enough to have the discussion and still not heavily drugged for pain. If you wait for "the right time," that time will never come because it is not easy to be direct in a society where directness is undervalued.

CONCLUSIONS

- *Open the discussion about death and fears by giving the sick person the confidence that you are really interested in what he or she has to say.*
- *Don't isolate the dying person either physically or emotionally.*
- *Don't wait till the last minute.*
- *The personal story (or the narration) gives meaning both to the dying person and to the listener.*

REFERENCES

1. "For a physician to provide exemplary care to patients experiencing fear of death, they must learn how to sit and support someone who is terrified of what lies before them. This involves emotional investment in a relationship despite one's own distress and doing everything possible to alleviate distress or pain. With this connection, structured support can be provided and the individual can be allowed to grieve for those they will miss, helping them to bear their suffering. Empathy and taking the time to be present and listen to the patient are some of the most important aspects" (Richard T. Penson, Rosamund A. Partridge, Muhammad A. Shah, David Giansiracusa, Bruce A. Chabner, & Thomas J. Lynch Jr., "Fear of Death," *Oncologist* 10 [2005]: 160–169).

2. "With death imminent, patients worry that no one is listening and fear dying with unnecessary pain and suffering. The SUPPORT study . . . suggests that these fears may be warranted . . . that . . . 46% of do-not-resuscitate (DNR) orders were written 2 days before death, and only 47% of physicians

knew patients' DNR preferences. Timely, sensitive discussions with seriously ill patients regarding medical, psychosocial, and spiritual needs at the end of life are both an obligation of and privilege for every physician. Physicians are also reluctant or unable to tell patients that they are likely to be approaching the end of their lives. . . . Consensus has evolved among clinicians that meaningful end-of-life options are usually offered too late. Fewer physicians agree as to the clinical markers signaling the time to initiate discussions" (Timothy E. Quill, M.D., "Initiating End-of-Life Discussions with Seriously Ill Patients, Addressing the 'Elephant in the Room,' " *Journal of the American Medical Association* 284 [2000]: 2502–2507).

7

The Silent Stage

∽

ENCOURAGING THE BEREAVED
TO EXPRESS THEMSELVES

"EVERY WEEK I would go and meet with Dr. Levi for half an hour. I would scream and cry, pound my fists on his desk, pull out my hair and swear. Then I would go out again to meet the world. Those sessions allowed me to remain sane." He looked down in silence, then raised his head, looked at the audience with wet eyes, and said, "Dr. Levi saved my life."

The man who spoke these impassioned words was an AIDS patient in his early thirties named John. He was virile looking, handsome, and muscular—not exactly your picture of someone with a life-threatening disease. The setting was a class of medical students in a course called "Breaking Bad News."

John said that when he was told that he was HIV positive, he felt like he had been hit by a truck. He knew he couldn't tell anyone that he had AIDS (which was how he saw it). He also knew he would never be able to bear the treatments and keep this knowledge completely to himself. So John asked Dr. Levi, who had given him the bad news, if he would be willing to meet with him for half an hour once a week until he could tell someone else about his disease. Dr. Levi agreed. It took John three years to tell someone else about the AIDS. During those three years, John would meet regularly with Dr. Levi.

This is how John described those meetings: "I would walk into Dr. Levi's office and sit down and cry, scream, tear out my hair. I would pound on the table and swear. I would do this for half an hour every week. Then I would stop, take a deep breath, and go out to meet the world. Dr. Levi saved my life."

Shortly thereafter, John left the auditorium, and Dr. Levi came to the stage, clearly overcome, shaking his head and shocked. This is what he said: "I am astonished! I am shocked. Yes, John was and is my patient. Yes, he asked to meet with me for half an hour a week until he could tell someone else about his disease. Yes, we met for three years. During those sessions, John never said a word! He didn't cry, he didn't scream, he didn't swear or pull his hair. I sat through those sessions feeling completely helpless. He would come in and sit down. There would be silence for half an hour every week. I felt like I was letting him down. He couldn't open up to me. I felt like a failure."

I spoke to Dr. Levi later and asked him, "Dr. Levi, is it possible that you sat three years in meetings with this man and didn't try to find out why he wasn't speaking?"

"I tried and tried, every way I knew to get him to talk or even to yell or cry, but nothing worked. After a while, I realized that this silence is what he wants. But until I heard him speak in your class, I didn't understand what he felt was happening in these meetings."

Why was Dr. Levi so successful? Because despite the fact that John didn't say a word, Dr. Levi let him have the stage. Usually, when we make a mistake, it is not because we are listening too much but because we are talking too much. In communication with the griever, there is never room for more than one on the stage. This means if you are talking, you are not listening. If you are really listening, you are not talking. You either take the stage or relinquish it to someone else.

The stage is more tempting for people to take than almost anything else because we receive it so infrequently. Therefore, even very reticent people are tempted to take the stage when it's given generously.

In my experience, there are only two ways to give the stage to someone. One way is by open-ended questions, for example, "How did you feel when you heard that you were HIV positive?" as opposed to closed questions that require a short answer, for example, "Did you feel bad when you heard you were HIV positive?" The second, and more difficult, way is through silence. You step off the stage and allow the other person to take it.

What happens when the person we give the stage to uses it for silence? We usually become uncomfortable and try to fill in the "empty" space. The problem here is that the silence is not always empty, as we see in John's story. Usually after receiving bad news, or another type of trauma, there is tremendous noise and confusion in the mind of the receiver. Thoughts come at great speed and intensity, and anything from the outside is experienced as interference. (This issue is dealt with again in chapter 9, "Decision to Live".) In general, there is no reason to be afraid of silence. Silence is an excellent way to give the stage to someone else. We need to look at what we are given without voice.

What is the significance of giving over the stage to the griever? In this case, John was grieving his loss of health and the other ramifications of his disease, such as being ostracized from society, lowered chances of raising a family, and living with the threat of death. He needed a place to express himself. His mode of expression was silence, sitting in a room with the only other person he knew who knew the truth. He could feel an outflow of all his frustration, rage, and pain without expressing it.

What really transpired in that room for three years? Was there total silence? Was there screaming and crying? Was it something in between? This is unimportant. What really happened, happened inside these two men—together, yet separate, in the same room once a week, half an hour, for three years.

John was very fortunate in his choice. He found a physician who was willing to give him a stage that he so desperately needed. When we give the stage to pain, we give it to the griever to do what he likes with it. It's his stage. It's his story. It's his life and death. We are just visitors. He can be an orator or a mime. The choice is his. How can we know whether it is effective? John returned to Dr. Levi's office every week for three years. Something must have been happening.

CONCLUSIONS

- *In communicating with the griever, remember that the stage is big enough just for one.*
- *Giving the stage can be accomplished through silence or questions.*
- *Allowing persons to express themselves, whether verbally or through silence, is important to facilitate grieving.*
- *Silence is a powerful tool, although difficult to use.*

REFERENCES

1. "Silence is an important aspect of human interaction, but is often experienced with discomfort and quickly filled with words. While quantitative parameters of silence such as timing and duration are easily recognized, qualitative experiential aspects are much more difficult to identify and describe. Emotions are experiential and complex, having antecedents in personal history, but words used to describe emotions are generally inadequate and simplistic. Silence is a useful experiential medium in which to identify and work with emotions. It is necessary to recognize what is being communicated by silence in each silence. This paper explores types of silences encountered in clinical work, and techniques to deal with them, avoiding symbolized language and technical terms of individual schools of psychotherapy" (G. Martyres, "On Silence: A Language for Emotional Experience," *Australian and New Zealand Journal of Psychiatry* 29 [1995]: 118–123).

2. "This research attempted to quantify specific behaviors in the physician's initial interviewing style and relate them to patients' perception of satisfaction. Twenty-seven percent of the variance

(*p* less than .01) in the satisfaction scores of initial interviews were explained by three aspects of a physician's language style: (a) use of silence or reaction time latency between speakers in an interview" (P. A. Rowland-Morin & J. G. Carroll, "Verbal Communication Skills and Patient Satisfaction: A Study of Doctor-Patient Interviews," *Evaluation and the Health Professions* 13 [1990]: 168–185).

3. "Listening and learning from the patient guides us as we acknowledge much of the mystery that still surrounds the dying process. Rarely is there a simple or right answer. An empathetic response to suffering patients is the best support. Support is vital in fostering the adjustment of patients. A silent presence may prove more helpful than well-meant counsel for many patients" (R. T. Penson, R. A. Partridge, M. A. Shah, D. Giansiracusa, B. A. Chabner, & T. J. Lynch Jr., "Fear of Death," *Oncologist* 10 [2005]: 160–169).

Where Is Safe?

⌒

Repercussions of Sibling Death

A YOUNG GIRL from the village came nervously into the open door. "Excuse me, I didn't want to disturb you. I am so sorry for your loss." The grieving parents looked up from where they sat clasping each other's hands on the couch, faces mottled from grief.

"Um, I, well, your little boy is sitting in the middle of the road crying and, um, I was afraid that a car might come and . . . " she paused helplessly. The parents jumped from their seats and ran out the door to the street, where, in the center of a bend in the road, their three-year-old son sat curled up crying. "My brother is dead. My brother is dead."

His startled parents lifted him up, cried with him, and held him close. "But, Yaya, you can't sit here, baby. You could get hurt. You know you are not allowed in the street alone."

"I don't care. My brother is dead, my brother is dead," he sobbed.

His brother, Paul, had been killed in a battle in Lebanon.

Three years later, Yaya was crying in his bed at night when his mother, Toni, came in to see what was wrong. She sat down beside him on the bed and stroked his hair. "Yaya, honey, why are you crying?"

" 'fraid!"

"What are you afraid of?"

"I'm 'fraid that you and dad will die before I go to the army." He sobbed, "I'm afraid no one will be here to tell me where in the army I will be safe."

Toni held him in her arms and called his father into the room. "Yaya is crying, Roy. He is afraid. He is afraid that we will die and no one will be here to tell him what unit in the army will be safe for him. Roy, where in the army will be safe for Yaya to serve?"

"I think the intelligence unit will be a safe place for him."

"Could you write that on a piece of paper for him?"

Yaya's father sat down and carefully printed out the word in block letters and gave the paper to Yaya with a hug and kissed the top of his head. "Does this help?"

Yaya nodded sniffling, climbed down from Toni's lap, and opened the drawer in the little night table next to his bed. He put the paper inside and closed it decisively. He looked at his parents, smiled a shaky smile, and climbed into bed.

"Are you okay, sweet baby?" his mother asked as she tucked him in and stroked his head.

"Yes." He smiled and closed his eyes. In a moment he was asleep.

The death of a child with small surviving siblings presents us with a problem not frequently found in grievers of other ages. Developmental issues permeate the grief.

Levels of understanding about the nature of death differ with age and with personal loss history. It is generally recognized that there are four aspects to understanding death: inevitability, irreversibility, causality, and totality. Many adults don't comprehend all of these concepts, but they are a way of measuring understanding.

Totality is probably the most confusing of these concepts and yet the most obvious in measurement. Totality means that the dead are actually dead; they don't eat, speak, play, breathe, and so on. In the language of small children, you can frequently hear the opposite: for example, "G'ma is in her coffin playing video games."

One of the things frequently seen in siblings that are younger than the child that died is a fear of reaching the same age of the deceased child at the time of death. This is particularly noticeable in same-sex siblings. This age can come closely following the death. It can also come decades later when we no longer expect to see significant repercussions of the grief. Why are these children afraid to reach this "dangerous" age? Because in their experience in the family, children don't survive past this age. The child is frequently afraid that he will also die and possibly by a death similar to that of the sibling. Most children under the age of eleven don't know that they can die. However, in a family where the death of a child has already occurred, the sense of safety and security is severely compromised, and the children know with a real knowing that they can also die and that their parents cannot necessarily protect them from death.

Under age eleven a child's whole support system is his parents. Yaya already knows that his parents have "failed to protect his brother," but as a small child, his options are few for other protection. So he is asking them in their "wisdom" to give him information that may be lost if they die. The main point here is that this child knows in a very practical way that death exists. Moreover, death exists for him and his family.

At this time Yaya needs an immediate answer to his question so he won't have to wait in suspense till he goes to the army. His parents cannot guarantee that they will not die before Yaya goes into the army, and they cannot promise what they cannot deliver. However, they can give him information that will make him feel safer in the interim. Even if the child doesn't understand the answer completely, if he receives an answer, this will allow him the opportunity to ask questions later as they come up.

What we really need to remember is that the relatively short attention span of children requires short direct answers to their questions. A child's concrete way of thinking demands practical answers.

Under age eleven and even frequently after that age, the child's thinking is almost exclusively egocentric. It is confined in attitude or interest to his own needs or affairs. In this case, Yaya's fears are both that he will die in the army and that his parents will die before they can "protect" him.

Many times a parent's answer to Yaya's fear, "I'm afraid that you and dad will die," would be "I won't die," which is a lie. Lying undermines a child's trust in his parents. In addition, the child knows this answer to be false because of the death that has already occurred in the family. A good approach is to answer the question that is asked on an honest, practical level. It is a tough challenge to come up with a practical and honest response to such a fear. Therefore, Yaya's father said, "I think the intelligence unit would be a safe place for you." Another possible honest answer to the question would be "Yaya, because Paul was killed, you will not go to a combat unit in the army, so you will be safer."

How do we know that the real question was answered for the child? We know by his response. He said yes, and he acted; he put the note in a safe place, and he went to sleep. The fact that his parents didn't sidestep his first question will allow him to address other questions about death or about the death of his brother more directly in the future. Generally, after a storm there is a lot of dead wood floating on the pond; you clean off what is on top first, then the deeper things float to the surface, and you can see what should be dealt with next.

If there is any doubt about the meaning, don't guess, don't assume; ask simple direct questions until the child's question becomes clear. And then answer in the most practical way you can. Check to see if this answer is acceptable to the child, as Roy did when he asked Yaya, "Does this help?" Philosophy and long answers are generally not good tools for communicating with small children.

CONCLUSIONS

- *Children are practical and need practical answers.*
- *Answer the question that is asked.*
- *If the question is not clear, ask for clarification.*
- *Don't lie to children.*
- *Expect long-term repercussions of sibling death.*

REFERENCES

1. "Unfortunately, there have been no longitudinal studies of bereaved children. Retrospective studies have suggested an increased vulnerability to adult psychiatric disorder, most notably depression. The long term risks of bereavement in childhood are associated with inadequate physical and emotional care, particularly after the loss of a mother. Certainly, the outcome for a child is strongly related to the way that adult carers are able to cope with their own grief and the changes to their lives, especially when bereavement is brought about by disaster or war. Children and adults who are bereaved by catastrophic events are particularly at risk of psychiatric disorders. Distress and long term sequelae can be lessened by early intervention" (D. Black, "Childhood Bereavement" [Editorial], *British Medical Journal* 312 [1996]: 1496).

9

Deciding to Live

∽

IMPORTANT DECISIONS
NEED CONSCIOUS THOUGHT

HER FIRSTBORN, MICHAEL, at twenty-eight, had been a young father who gave her her first grandchild. She had three other children, all strong, tall, and athletic. One would be in the army soon. Three others had already passed that daily danger and she those sleepless nights, successfully. Now they only had to serve in reserve army duty one month a year.

And here was Michael, with a promising future ahead of him, a sweet wife, and a small child. It happened late last night. Michael and his wife were at a disco, dancing, when suddenly, for no apparent reason, Michael fell, like a tree, holding his chest. In moments, he was dead. The ambulance came, the local clinic rushed to the scene, tried to resuscitate, but no chance; it was over. When the death was investigated, it was found that Michael had suffered a massive heart attack.

Within twelve hours of his death, according to the Israeli custom of the soonest possible burial, Michael was to be buried.

Now Tamar, Michael's mother, found herself hospitalized for the first time since her youngest child's birth. It was twelve noon. Michael's funeral would begin in two hours. She would not be able to attend. She had had her first heart attack within hours of Michael's death. She was wired to monitors and an IV. I was sitting beside her bed holding her hand.

We were silent. She was pale and looked as though she had taken a physical beating. After some time she looked at me. Both of our eyes filled again with tears. I spoke for the first time since I had come. "Tamar, you have shown that you want to die. You have even shown that you are capable of dying." I paused for a moment. She continued to look at me steadily through her tears. "I would like to ask you not to let your body make this decision for you. Think about what you really want and then decide. Do you want to live, or do you want to die? Make the decision with your mind, not your body." She continued to look at me for another moment, and then her eyes wandered away. She went to her "personal library," her history, everything she knew and thought about herself, her culture, her experiences. She examined what she had lost and what remained. She weighed the pluses and minuses in order to make her decision. After about fifteen minutes of silence, her eyes returned to mine, and she said, "I have decided to live." I smiled and said, "I am very glad."

Even in the most difficult times, perhaps especially in the most difficult times, we need to make decisions with our minds, not our bodies. Making an active decision to live after horrible trauma is often the first step to recovery, even while the aftershocks of the trauma are still fresh. If we wait too long to make this decision, our "nondecision" can solidify and become difficult to identify and break out of. In Tamar's case, a lack of an immediate decision could cause the threat to her life to become even more profound.

Do we want the traumatized person to live? If we are helping someone we care about, then chances are good that we do want them to live. If we are professionals in the field, we know that most traumatized and bereaved people do recover from trauma or bereavement and successfully return to rich, albeit different, lives. People who make life-changing or life-endangering decisions based on the tremendous pain they are feeling in the first few months following the trauma or bad news are making decisions on the basis of a fallacy. This fallacy is the belief "I will forever feel as horrible as I feel this moment." We know that generally speaking, the intensity of this pain will change over time. On a rare occasion, it may also become worse, but it usually lessens.

Is it entirely up to the individual whether or not he will live or die? Not entirely, but there are other options. We all know people who are the "walking dead." Physically they live, but they have emotionally absented themselves from life. Whether this decision was made actively or passively, they have chosen not to live.

After a trauma, regardless of whether the person is speaking or not, his thoughts have a tendency to be crowded and confused, coming at great speed and numbers. Sometimes when we try to send a message, by speaking, to the traumatized person, we are not, in fact, able to communicate with him. Why? Because no one is there to receive this message. The person is absent. One way to be sure a sighted person can hear you is to watch their eyes. Normally, when we are reflecting on something other than what is happening in front of us, we avert our gaze. This averted gaze frequently signifies introspection. When our attention is turned inward, particularly after trauma, we are not available to receive additional outside information. If we try to communicate with the traumatized person verbally, this can cause two types of communication disruption.

First, we believe we have communicated something that, in fact, has not been received. If this communication is important, then the person we are talking to will not hear it again because we believe the information has already been passed on to them. Incorrect assumptions about what they know and don't know will be made on that basis. One of the frequent causes of miscommunication occurs when we think we are sending a message, but, in fact, we are not because no one is available to receive the message.

Second, the traumatized individual needs time to process what has happened. Pulling them out of or attempting to pull them out of their inner reflection is intrusive and unwise. In counseling situations, people have frequently reported, "I heard her babbling at my side [the nurse] and just wanted to scream at her, 'Shut up so I can think!' " or "He [the doctor] wouldn't stop talking! I wanted to slap him!"

The best way to use this information is to stop speaking when the eyes travel and wait until they return to you. When they do return, wait for about five seconds before speaking. This is to offer an opportunity for the other person to speak first. If he or she does not speak after this pause, I usually resume the conversation by asking, "Where were you just now?" Usually the answer to this question is the most significant part of the conversation.

CONCLUSIONS

- *Following trauma, it is frequently necessary for the traumatized individual to make a clear decision to live.*
- *When the traumatized person's eyes travel, do not speak. When the eyes return, wait for four to five seconds before speaking.*
- *Important decisions need conscious thought.*

REFERENCES

1. "Eye contact plays a central role in interpersonal relations. The eyes preface most new relationships, overshadowing other sensory inputs while transmitting a wide assortment of emotional cues. Visual behavior may at times prove decisive in assuring survival, in amorous encounters, and in clarifying interpersonal motives. Ocular performance, a final common pathway for many social, cultural and emotional determinants, is a crucial factor in defining relationships and in allowing reciprocal influences to be exchanged as persons relate. In psychiatric patients, ocular behavior may provide clues to diagnosis. A common finding in such persons is gaze aversion, a social avoidance phenomenon which indicates a desire to attenuate the interpersonal experience and thereby decrease anxiety" (G. W. Grumet, "Eye Contact: The Core of Interpersonal Relatedness," *Psychiatry* 46 [1983]: 172–180).

2. "Gaze direction is a vital communicative channel through which people transmit information to each other. By signaling the locus of social attention, gaze cues convey information about the relative importance of objects, including other people, in the

environment. For the most part, this information is communicated via patterns of gaze direction, with gaze shifts signaling changes in the objects of attention" (M. F. Mason, E. P. Tatkow, & C. N. Macrae, "The Look of Love: Gaze Shifts and Person Perception," *Psychological Science* 16 [2005]: 236–239).

3. "When gaze direction matches the underlying behavioral intent (approach-avoidance) communicated by an emotional expression, the perception of that emotion would be enhanced (i.e., shared signal hypothesis). Specifically, . . . (a) direct gaze would enhance the perception of approach-oriented emotions (anger and joy) and (b) averted eye gaze would enhance the perception of avoidance-oriented emotions (fear and sadness)" (R. B. Adams Jr. & R. E. Kleck, "Effects of Direct and Averted Gaze on the Perception of Facially Communicated Emotion," *Emotion* (Washington, D.C.) 5 [2005]: 3–11).

10

Who's Next?

~

TAKING CHILDREN TO FUNERALS: WHEN, WHAT AGE, HOW

NAOMI DECIDED SHE would take the girls to the funeral after all. It is true that they were very young, four and six, but she was sure that the funeral would be a low-key, quiet affair. What better way to give her children an opportunity to say goodbye to their great-grandmother and also to be part of the grieving group and gain an understanding of death and their culture?

Naomi knew there would be no overt emotion or drama at this funeral. Great-grandma Henrietta was ninety-nine at the time of her death. Despite her considerable contributions earlier in life, in the later part of her life, she had been a difficult, critical, and sick woman. There would be no crying.

Naomi walked with the girls following the car bearing Henrietta's coffin on the way to the small graveyard. They were part of a sizable group of about a hundred from her community going to the funeral.

They entered the graveyard. The grave had already been dug and there was a large pile of dirt next to it with several shovels standing in it.

Naomi went to the side with a clear view of the grave with her daughters, Hope and Dawn. She squatted down beside them and began to quietly answer questions and explain the proceedings. Henrietta's plain pine coffin was taken from the car and carried to the lip of the grave. Belts were placed around it, and it was gently lowered into the open grave.

The belts were slid out from around the coffin and out of the grave. Men from the village went to the pile of dirt, took shovels, and began to fill the grave quietly. The first shovelful of dirt made a soft hollow thud as it fell on the coffin. Naomi glanced anxiously at Hope's and Dawn's small faces waiting for a response. Dawn partially turned toward her mother, her eyes glued to the scene in front of her.

"Why are they putting dirt on Great-Gramma's coffin?"

"Well, honey, our friends help us to bury our dead, and we help them to bury their dead."

"Mom, can I put a shovel of dirt into the grave?"

"Honey, you are a bit small for a shovel; they are heavy. Maybe you want to take a handful of dirt and put it in?"

Dawn nodded and solemnly went to the pile of dirt, took a handful, and went to the lip of the grave and dropped it in.

She came back to Naomi. "Mommy, can I put a shovel of dirt in next year?" "Depends on our luck, baby."

The funeral continued, eulogy, placing flowers, greeting the mourners. The girls followed the proceedings avidly.

At the conclusion of the funeral, those who had come from afar were invited to light refreshments before they began their drive home. People sat around the room talking. Hope sat on her grandmother's lap. She had always been a speaker, setting forth her views as oratory. Hope began, her small voice piping up, clearly demanding the attention of all who sat near. "I have three grandmothers: Gramma Faith, she's dead; Gramma Henrietta, she's dead; and Gramma Eve [on whose knees she sat], she will soon die." A shocked silence followed by laughter ensued. Everyone laughed except Gramma Eve.

Small children view death in a linear fashion. In Hope's experience, grandfathers, parents, siblings didn't die; only grandmothers died. Her expectation reflects her personal experience.

Why were Hope and Dawn at the funeral? A funeral is a family event. As with a wedding, the whole family should be present. Anyone who is not present will feel left out in some way. Today or tomorrow when looking back on the event, the child may ask, "Why wasn't I there?"

Frequently, we leave children out of funerals or formal mourning ceremonies in order to "protect" them from pain and sadness. In truth, it is hard to know how to cope with children in the shadow of death. But avoidance of children's participation in the mourning rituals doesn't protect them in the long run; it isolates them. If they don't participate, they are not part of the grieving group despite the fact that they will have to bear the absence of the deceased family member. They miss out, if not included, on seeing the impact their loved one had on others, outside of family members, who will miss the deceased. They do not receive support and expressions of sympathy and care that are customarily given in the formal mourning period. The reason these customs continue to exist is that we feel they help. Would we deny this help to our children?

Additionally, the death of a loved one is usually accompanied by guilt feelings. The cause of these guilt feelings may be some minor slight, or a more difficult relationship or event in the relationship. Not allowing a child to participate in formal mourning rituals may exacerbate the guilt. The child often reasons that dad didn't want him at his funeral because he didn't like him, or because he fought with him some time ago. Sometimes these same children come to my clinic years later as adults with feelings of heavy guilt associated with their parents' deaths.

Much of the child's understanding of the funeral and the formal mourning period is gleaned from the person who accompanies the child or the person who explains the proceedings to the child in advance. Naomi knew the funeral would pass without event and so chose to explain it to the girls on site. In the case of sudden, unexpected death, it is better to explain, in detail, what happens at a funeral ahead of time because this type of funeral tends to have more dramatic expressions of grief and shock. Knowledge is something we hang on to when facing new situations, like reading a map when we need to find our way around.

CONCLUSIONS

- *Children frequently think in a linear fashion, expecting same role relatives to die the way that Hope expected Gramma Eve to die.*
- *It is important to take children to funerals and not to send them to school or kindergarten during the formal mourning period.*
- *It is worthwhile to explain to children what will happen and what they are expected to do at the funeral or formal mourning rituals. This can be done ahead of time, and should be done ahead of time, if possible, in the event of sudden, unexpected death.*

REFERENCES

1. "When death occurs, young children in particular may need the concrete experience of seeing the parent after death. Bereaved adults find it particularly difficult to help a child in this way, and the general practitioner could offer to accompany the child. Similarly, children benefit from attending the funeral but need some protection from the raw expressed grief that may be shown at that time. Attending in the company of someone less affected by the death than the immediate relatives is desirable. This could be the child's teacher or someone from the family practice with whom he is familiar. . . . Children are rarely prepared for the death of a parent or a sibling, and yet we know from studies of bereaved adults that mourning is aided by a foreknowledge of the imminence and inevitability of death. Children who are forewarned have lower levels of anxiety than those who are not, even within the same family" (D. Black, "Bereavement in Childhood," *British Medical Journal* 316 [1998]: 931–933).

11

The Worst Death

⤚

THE DIFFERENCE BETWEEN
LOSING A PARENT AND LOSING A CHILD

"SO HOW HAVE you been sleeping during the past week?" I asked.

"Fine."

"And your eating habits?"

"The same."

"Okay, and . . . "

"You think I don't know they are dead, don't you?"

"Well, there is a strong chance that you don't really get it yet."

I was talking to a fifteen-year-old boy, named Joel, who had lost his entire family, two months earlier, in a terrorist bombing at a family wedding in a restaurant. He had gone outside about a block away to secretly smoke a cigarette and was the only survivor of three generations.

He was quiet for a few minutes, looking down at his hands folded between his legs. He looked up.

"How long will it take for me to understand that they are all dead?"

I paused. "I can't really be sure. Usually after the sudden, unexpected death of someone who is important to you, it takes somewhere around three months to understand that the person is dead. With your situation, when so many people have died, it is hard to tell when the understanding will come."

He nodded, then asked, "Why does it take so long?"

"Well," I said, gathering my thoughts, "physically, death actually happens in a fraction of a second. But our emotional connection to our loved ones is not so easy to deal with. We begin to understand when they consistently don't come home every day at the time they used to. They are never in that chair again where they used to sit. They don't call or continue building the relationship in any way, and the emptiness sets in. It isn't the same as the mental knowledge that they are dead. We can say the words as soon as we hear them, but we don't understand what they mean. Grief is slow. It's really a dinosaur in modern life. You can get a meal in three minutes from a fast food place, in a minute you can get any information you want from the Internet, but pregnancy and grief still take a long time."

He looked down at his hands again and looked up. "When I realize what happened, will I lose my mind?" I waited a moment before answering. "You may want to lose your mind, but you will not."

We sat in silence for a few minutes, and then Joel asked, "Is this death the worst death that anyone can go through?"

"Well," I paused, "experts say that the death of the child is the worst death to deal with. But again, you lost so many people . . . I can't really say."

"Why would the death of a child be worse than what I am having to deal with?"

"This is an important question," I replied. "Give me a few minutes." I sat back in my chair and stopped looking at Joel for the first time during the meeting. I searched for an appropriate and honest answer. After about four minutes I sat forward again. Joel was still sitting waiting for me.

"Joel, you have sustained tremendous losses, your parents, siblings, grandparents, aunts and uncles and cousins. You have also sustained all the associated losses of support, home, and hearth. You have lost many things, but you have not lost the future. The death of a child is the loss of the future."

Joel nodded, looked down, and smiled at his hands. "Yep, they couldn't take my future away from me."

CONCLUSIONS

- *Normal grief is a very long process—it takes a long time.*
- *One person's grief can be compared with another's grief, but don't lose sight of the person in front of you and his specific situation.*
- *You always have something to offer, no matter how inadequate you think it is—you may be the connection to life that the grieving person needs.*

REFERENCES

1. "Complicated grief, unlike normal or uncomplicated grief, is not a self-limited process that presumably starts with a stage of initial shock, moves on to a stage of acute somatic or emotional

discomfort and social withdrawal, and then ends with the acceptance of the loss and restoration of prebereavement levels of
functioning. Rather, complicated grief is the failure to return to
preloss levels of performance or states of emotional well-being.
For a considerable minority of bereaved persons, emotional and
behavioral disturbances persist and prevent the return to normal
functioning" (H. G. Prigerson, E. Frank, S. V. Kasl, C. F. Rey-
nolds III, B. Anderson, G. S. Zubenko, P. R. Houck, C. J.
George, & D. J. Kupfer, "Complicated Grief and Bereavement-
Related Depression as Distinct Disorders: Preliminary Empirical
Validation in Elderly Bereaved Spouses," *American Journal of Psychiatry* 152 [1995]: 22–30).

2. "In order to share one's emotions, one needs others who
are willing to listen. Measures of perceived social support reflect
the availability of others to whom one can disclose one's emotions. The assumption that support from family and friends is
one of the most important moderators of bereavement outcome is widely accepted among bereavement researchers and
practitioners. . . . Social support can play a role at two different
points in the causal chain that links stress to illness: social support
can influence stress appraisal and/or it can result in 'inhibition
of maladjustive and facilitation of adjustive responses.' . . . Thus,
the knowledge that one can call on the support of friends and
family members, and that one does not have to face a lonely
future, may help to soften the blow of the loss and buffer one
against the deleterious effects of bereavement. More relevant in
the context of this article is the second pathway, namely the
facilitation of coping through the inhibition of maladjustive and
the facilitation of adjustive counter responses. Accordingly, even
if the availability of social support should fail to buffer the individual against the impact of bereavement by attenuating stress
appraisal, the emotional support from family and friends should
facilitate grief work by making it possible for the bereaved to

express their feelings and reactions to the death of a loved one. Thus, by encouraging the expression of emotion, the provision of social support could accelerate recovery and promote long-term adjustment" (W. Stroebe, H. Schut, & M. S. Stroebe, "Grief Work, Disclosure and Counseling: Do They Help the Bereaved?" *Clinical Psychology Review* 25 [2005]: 395–414).

12

The Last to Know

$\backsim$

THE INDIVIDUAL'S RIGHT TO KNOW

"WE HAVE A PROBLEM," the doctor said as we sat with the staff in a clinic in a small village.

"What's the problem?" I asked.

"Abel Cohen was admitted to the hospital for exploratory surgery at age forty-six. They opened him up and closed him immediately. You know what that means."

"Inoperable metastasized cancer? Is he dying?"

"Yes."

"So why did you call me today?"

"He is in the hospital. His wife told the neighbors, and now the whole village knows what he has. He is coming home tomorrow, and he is the only one who doesn't know."

"Go to the hospital and tell him," I said to the doctor.

"It's not that simple," he replied. "The surgeon there said I can't, and as long as the patient is in his territory and under his authority, I can't."

"Bring me Abel's wife," I replied.

Forty minutes later, Shoshie, Abel's wife, met with me in a room at the clinic.

"Tell me what happened with Abel."

Shoshie began with the pains Abel had begun to feel and how he had tried to ignore them for months till it was impossible to continue to ignore them. She continued the story through the doctor's appointments and the operation yesterday.

"Does he know?"

"No," she replied. "The surgeon said Abel would jump out the window to his death if we tell him."

"Tell me about your husband. What kind of a man is he?"

Shoshie proceeded to describe an industrious, ambitious, determined, bright man of many significant accomplishments both in the military and in civilian life.

"Would Abel want to know what is happening to him?"

"Abel always wants to know everything about everything. I think he would want to know."

"Can you go tell him?"

"No. The surgeon said he would commit suicide if I tell him."

"Abel will not commit suicide. At least not until he finds out everything about his disease."

"Then why did the surgeon say he would?"

"How many minutes did the surgeon see Abel while Abel was conscious?"

"Three or four."

"Abel will not commit suicide at this point."

"Then why did the surgeon say he would?"

"The surgeon thinks that that is what he himself would do if he had Abel's disease. It is not related to your husband."

"But how can I tell him?"

"You go into his room at the hospital and say, 'Abel, I think that you have the right to know everything about what you have. So, any questions you have, just ask me. If I have the answer I will tell you. If I don't have the answer, I will find it out.' Then stop talking and wait."

"What will he do?"

"He just had an operation. He will ask what they found. Be careful to use the word 'growth' or 'tumor' and not 'infection' or anything else."

"Then what?"

"Then he will ask the next logical question. Is the tumor cancer or not? You say cancer, and it is done. Four sentences and two words. This way he sets the pace, and he is in control of the conversation."

"Then what will he do?"

"He will say, 'I knew it.'"

Shoshie went to the hospital two hours later and then came to my clinic to tell me what had transpired. She said, "It happened as you said. And when he said, 'I knew it,' I was stunned! I am an atheist and only believe in what I can see. But suddenly I thought, 'Perhaps everyone knows when they are about to die in some type of spiritual, mysterious, otherworldly knowledge.' So I asked Abel, 'How did you know?' He said, 'My brother, whom I haven't spoken to in fourteen years, calls me at the hospital from South Africa. Everyone who comes to visit has red swollen eyes.'"

"Then why didn't you say anything?" Shoshie said she asked him.

"I felt I wasn't allowed. No one would look me in the eye. I felt ashamed and embarrassed."

When I first met Shoshie, it was important for me to hear her story. Shoshie's story is not the doctor's story, nor is it the surgeon's or anyone else's. Shoshie's story is her own. In order to understand what can be done, it is important to hear her story told her way, and she needs to know that I hear her story. Everyone has a story to tell about every event.

Because of the special husband-wife relationship, Shoshie probably knows Abel better than any of the professionals on the case. I would better understand Abel from her perspective than from anyone else's except for Abel himself, who was not available to talk at that time.

Unless otherwise notified by the individual in question, a sick person or patient deserves to know the truth at his own pace, not a pace someone else chooses for him, not a "protection" from the truth, which usually backfires into feelings of betrayal.

The life of the patient is his. No one can live it for him, and the choices about it remain his, even when he is ill. To make choices for himself, he needs relevant information. Choices made on the basis of deceit cannot be balanced choices. Most often, I suggest stating the willingness to answer any questions the dying person may have.

As in the case of the surgeon, when we try to make choices for other people, these choices are usually based on our own subjective reality, including our fears and doubts. These feelings that we sometimes assume to be universal are not universal but personal. Basing decisions that affect someone else on our personal biases is inaccurate and unhelpful.

CONCLUSIONS

- *Everyone has his or her own story, and we need to hear each story from the individual perspective.*
- *Everyone is entitled to hear the truth at his or her own pace.*
- *Transference of your fears to the person you are speaking to can cloud your judgment and vision.*

REFERENCES

1. "In their various forms, stories provide a means of organizing material about human behavior and events in the world. As individuals interpret human behavior, we give meaning to our experiences in the world by creating stories, making sense out of events, and explaining why people do what they do—invoking such notions as concern, value, belief, commitment, motive, and desire. Sociologists Berger and Luckman . . . emphasized the importance of stories in shaping social realities, showing how people's characteristic stories change as they move from one life event to another. The central role of story telling in human affairs is fundamental to our understanding of individuals. . . . From our perceptions of what has happened to us, we tell a story that reveals a narrative of events and evaluations of the experience. The resulting narrative is a text that has both a subtext and a context. The subtext can be thought of as the values and goals that are driving and shaping the narrative. The context is made

up of life experiences that filter the current interpretation. All three components—text, subtext, and context—are crucial to understanding the central theme of an individual's narrative and the decision-making processes associated with it" (A. J. Young & K. L. Rodriguez, "The Role of Narrative in Discussing End-of-life Care: Eliciting Values and Goals from Text, Context, and Subtext," *Health Communication* 19 [2006]: 49–59).

2. "The author [L. Grinberg] considers whether the reason for the variety and multiplicity of theories about the transference might lie in analysts' fears of its dangers. He reviews Freud's development of the concept from its origins, when it was seen as resistance, to its use as a fundamental instrument of the treatment and lays particular emphasis on its perception as a burden. . . . The author emphasizes the importance of the analyst's training and experience in enabling him to withstand the regressive onslaught of the patient's projections without resorting to theory-related or technical defensive measures. In his view, the transference is not in itself a resistance but may be used as such. The analyst must not interpret merely in order to get rid of the anxiety aroused in himself by the patient's regressive feelings" (L. Grinberg, "Is the Transference Feared by the Psychoanalyst?" *International Journal of Psychoanalysis* 78 [1997]: 1–14).

13

What Is Freedom?

◦—

THE UNIQUE PERSPECTIVE
OF THE INDIVIDUAL

JUDAH, TWENTY-FIVE, was on a trip abroad with Susan, twenty-two, his girlfriend of long standing. They were in a desolate area when they had a car accident.

Susan was seriously hurt with a head injury. Judah got out of the car unscathed (at least physically). It was hours before they could get any assistance and even longer before they reached a hospital. Susan was unable to communicate, and it was not clear whether she was aware of her surroundings.

Judah held onto hope through the next year while Susan was an inpatient in a rehabilitation hospital. He was so distressed at her condition, and so invested in his relationship with Susan, that he devoted all his time and energy to her recovery. Every day he visited her at the hospital, learning the physiotherapy exercises that were demanded of her, seeking the best care available for her, the best chances for recovery, the most advanced facilities.

Susan had become a different person. So had Judah. His own life ceased to exist. Judah wanted to do everything for her, and as a result Susan was doing less and less for herself.

It was never completely clear what Susan thought about all this. In addition to the physical abilities she had lost, she could barely speak. When other family members took shifts at the hospital, Susan's progress was more pronounced. But it was still very slow—excruciatingly slow. This pattern continued for over a year.

Judah began to meet with me to try to sort out his feelings. Gradually, he was encouraged to resume his own life. His first step was to get a job and reduce the number of hours that he spent at the hospital. After that, he needed to start looking into university preparation courses. He initially decided to study physiotherapy. But guilt, mixed with responsibility and dedication, prevented him from reducing the hours that he spent with Susan at the hospital.

At one stage, Judah decided he really needed to make money more quickly. But without a degree or profession, and with only the odd hours he could work between hospital visits, he had no chance for a high-paying job. In spite of much trepidation about leaving Susan, he finally decided to travel to the Far East for three months to sell "imitations" of brand-name products. He would set up a market stand and earn a lot of money in a short time. Judah assured me that although this kind of business was not legal, he was in no danger because it was a business that the local authorities ignored.

It was important that he go, not because of his money-making scheme, but because he desperately needed a break from caring for Susan. The physical distance between them would enable him to get a clearer perspective on his responsibilities toward others and himself.

Judah declared that he would be calling Susan at least once every day. Someone would put the phone next to her ear so she would be able to hear him. She herself still could not speak.

When he arrived at his destination, he made the necessary connections and obtained a market stand. He was told that a new "imitation" had hit the market, but it was still "hot" and was therefore risky to sell at the moment. Judah decided to take the risk with the "hot" new item and to even go out on a limb by tripling the size of his stand.

Shortly after he began to work, he was arrested and imprisoned. While not mistreated, he was allowed only one visitor a week, for an hour. He was not allowed to make any phone calls at all.

There was a "mobile library" wheeled around to the prisoners in their cells during the week. Of course, there were no books in his native Hebrew language, so Judah began reading voraciously in English (a required language in all Israeli schools). Ironically, he devoured mostly John Grisham courtroom dramas. His English improved dramatically.

Judah was imprisoned for three months altogether. He was not permitted to speak with Susan even once during that period. He had, however, a legitimate reason for his prolonged silence. He also had the fear of a much longer prison sentence hanging over his head.

When he returned to Israel, he called to set up an appointment. He was thinner and quieter than the last time he came. During our meeting he commented, "How strange—for many years I haven't felt the freedom that I felt while in jail." He then built a framework that would enable him to retain the freedom that he had obtained at no small price.

It was decided that the best schedule would be for Judah to be with Susan and help with her care only one morning a week. He would see her socially only one afternoon a week. He had discovered that during his imprisonment she had been well cared for without him. She had worked harder when he was less available to assist (or overassist) her in her exercises.

Words like "love," "peace," and "freedom" are ambiguous and hard to define. Most people would assume that a man in prison cannot be free, and yet this assumption is frequently wrong. Judah had been "a prisoner" in life, and through jail he was forced to step out of life to achieve a measure of "freedom."

With Judah, his limitations were physical: incarceration in a foreign jail. His freedom came through his own perception of his situation, meaning, and emotions. Moreover, the "reality" of his situation, as Judah perceived it and responded to it, could not be grasped through outside observation alone. It required hearing his personal narrative to understand it.

It was another year before we met again. I asked permission to use his prison story in this book. He looked down, smiled his slow smile, and shook his head in wonder. "It was such an amazing part of my life, that time in prison. I am sure it saved me years of mistakes." He looked up. "Can you imagine the odds against it having happened that way? Here was this tragedy. Then suddenly, from nowhere, comes this odd 'solution' to make me step out of my life and look at it. What are the odds against something like that happening?"

"What? Judah, you made it happen. You chose the 'hot' item, you chose to triple the size of the market stand. You arranged that flight into freedom."

He looked up, surprised, and then smiled again, "Yes, I guess I did. You can't always know where your freedom will be found."

CONCLUSIONS

- *The "obvious" truth is not always true.*
- *The subjective reality is contained in the narrative.*
  You need the narrative to see the person.

REFERENCES

1. "Firstly, [narrative as a linguistic form] has a finite and longitudinal time sequence—that is, it has a beginning, a series of unfolding events, and (we anticipate) an ending. . . . Secondly, it presupposes both a narrator and a listener whose different viewpoints affect how the story is told. Thirdly, the narrative is concerned with individuals; rather than simply reporting what they do or what is done to them it concerns how those individuals feel and how people feel about them. . . . The narrative also provides information that does not pertain simply or directly to the unfolding events. The same sequence of events told by another person to another audience might be presented differently without being any less 'true.' This is an important point. In contrast with a list of measurements or a description of the outcome of an experiment, there is no self-evident definition of what is relevant or what is irrelevant in a particular narrative. The choice

of what to tell and what to omit lies entirely with the narrator and can be modified, at his or her discretion, by the questions of the listener" (T. Greenhalgh & B. Hurwitz, "Education and Debate: Narrative-Based Medicine, Why Study Narrative?" *British Medical Journal* 318 [1999]: 48–50).

14

The Mailman

LEARN AND PASS THE KNOWLEDGE ON

HIS MOTHER WEPT QUIETLY into the crumpled tissue in her hand. "And the nurse, my friend, came to me and said, 'Don't worry, I didn't let strangers touch him at all. I cleaned his body and prepared him. I was the last one to touch your son Aviv before his burial.'" She moaned and held her head tightly between clenched fists. "Why wasn't I the last one to touch my son?"

This was Smadar's repeated woe, reiterated frequently at our weekly meetings. Her son was only three at the time of his death from a fatal respiratory (breathing) disease. This disease had stalked him since birth, carrying a diagnosis predicting certain death at a young age. It had been six months since Aviv's death.

Now I was facing a different kind of problem. I was counseling another couple with a small child suffering from the same disease; the same inevitable outcome would be confronting them in the near future. Should I warn them? Should I tell them? If I tell them and they do not have the strength to prepare their child for burial, will it mean that they will feel worse than if I had said nothing?

I thought about this other couple, Judith and Alan. What would they do with this information if I were to give it to them? Could I speak so plainly about the child's burial and body preparation while the child was still alive? And if not, then what? Would this mournful refrain of Smadar's become Judith's also? What was my obligation? I thought of the quote "Do not withhold good from those to whom it is due when it is in the power of your hand to do so" (Proverbs 3:27, NKJV). But was this good? I reminded myself that Judith had always asked for every tool or information that could possibly help her, both with her son's disease and with the family's coping. She had been in control most of the time all of her life and was grasping for control over any detail. It was clear. I would speak to them about this.

We met in their tastefully decorated living room for the meeting that day. They greeted me with the traditional cup of coffee, and we sat down to talk on two sofas at right angles to each other. Alan sat beside Judith.

"I have something very, very hard to discuss with you today. It is something that might help you or might also hurt you. I need your permission to open this subject before I continue." I waited.

Judith and Alan looked at each other. Judith set her jaw and prepared herself for yet another blow in this exhausting ordeal. They both looked at me expectantly.

"Because you have a nurse that is helping you at home . . ." I paused, then began again. "Another client of mine had a young child who died. Her child's body was prepared for burial by the clinic nurse, who was a friend. The mother always talks about how hard it is for her to know that she didn't prepare her child herself. You need to know that when May dies, you do not have to let strangers prepare her body for burial. You can do it yourself with the nurse's observation. This way, if you want to and if you have the strength, you can be the last ones to touch May's body before she is buried."

Alan covered his face with his hands. Judith looked at me, eyes full of tears. She swallowed a few times. She tried to speak, swallowed again and spoke in a voice heavy with emotion, "Thank you."

About two months later, May died. Judith called me. "It is over," she said. I said, "I'm coming." May was laid out on the bed. She looked like Snow White, beautiful and peaceful.

The next morning I arrived in the village for the funeral and went directly to the family home. Judith greeted me at the door with a cry, throwing herself into my arms. This was very unusual. Our contact, which had been long term, had never involved any physical contact. She said, "I don't know how I will ever be able to thank you. I will never be able to thank you."

I came in and sat with her on the rug. She said, "When May died, I held her and held her. I felt I could never let her go. It had been so long since I was able to hold her without all the breathing machinery. Then I stood up with her and made her a bubble bath. She loved bubble baths. I washed her small body, I combed her hair, I brushed her teeth. I dressed her and even put on a new diaper. I wrapped her up, and I—by myself—I put her in the small coffin that had been prepared for her. I kissed her and closed the lid."

Later that week, I had a meeting with Smadar. She said to me, "Did you know there was another small child in Israel who recently died from the same disease that took our Aviv?"

"Really?" I replied.

"Yes," she said, "and I know that you know, and I know that you have been counseling them."

"Okay," I replied.

She continued, "I know you can't talk about it, but I just need to ask you one question."

"Ask," I replied.

Smadar's eyes filled with tears. "Did you tell them to be the last ones to touch their child?"

I looked at her and spoke quietly. "I did. And they were the last to touch their child. And this was a gift to them, from you, because I never could have known the importance without you."

She let a sob escape from her lips. "At least that . . . at least that."

A large part of my job is that of a "mailman." It is to move information from one client to another.

When we go into our chosen work (regardless of what it might be), we go in with a basic understanding of what the job entails. This basic understanding may be the minimum we need to function in the work. It is on the job that we really learn what must be done in different situations that we encounter.

In any situation between two human beings, two worlds are meeting. In a counseling situation, there are two experts in the room. The counselor is an expert in his or her field, and the person receiving counseling is an expert in his or her own life, history, defense, and coping mechanisms. The meeting works best when both areas of expertise are respected and taken into account. When this happens, there is an enormous amount of learning available.

In work with people, we learn from the people we have contact with. With each encounter, there is something to be learned on the negative or positive side—or sometimes both. As we witness and become a part of different human situations, we gain knowledge that waits to be put to use at the appropriate moment. It's like working a jigsaw puzzle; we try to determine which piece of information will fit where.

My colleague and friend Eric Cassell put it this way: "We are always trying to protect our clients or loved ones or patients from hurts—both literal and figurative. Sometimes we don't tell them terribly painful things because we are afraid it will hurt them. Leaving out for the moment that we are also afraid for ourselves in the saying of the awful thing. The question is usually: what is the greater protection: telling them or not telling them? This too one learns from direct experience with people; they can tolerate a lot more than you initially think, and then be better for it. Except, sometimes it isn't true; they cannot handle it. It isn't just them, after all you are there also and the combination of them and you usually makes them (and you) stronger than them (or you) alone" (personal correspondence, May 2005).

CONCLUSIONS

- *When giving someone difficult information, first ask the person's permission so that they can prepare themselves.*
- *Books and classes are not enough; we can and should learn from every encounter we have both personally and in the field. We would never know what to do if the people we take care of were not our teachers.*
- *People are usually very resilient and can handle a lot more than we, or they, think they can.*
- *Sometimes one needs to make a decision about what would be more helpful for the person we are talking to. It is a calculated risk, based on our already acquired knowledge of the person. It isn't always an easy decision and should be weighed carefully.*

REFERENCES

1. "Steps 2 and 3 of SPIKES are points in the interview where you implement the axiom 'before you tell, ask.' That is, before discussing the medical findings, the clinician uses open-ended questions to create a reasonably accurate picture of how the patient perceives the medical situation—what it is and whether it is serious or not" (W. F. Baile, R. Buckman, R. Lenzia, G. Glober, E. A. Beale, & A. P. Kudelka, "SPIKES—A Six-Step Protocol for Delivering Bad News: Application to the Patient with Cancer," *Oncologist* 5 [2000]: 302–311).

15

I Want Attention

∽

CLASSROOM INTERVENTION AFTER SUICIDE

IN THE ROOM there were low chairs and pillows positioned against all four walls with about twenty-five thirteen-year-olds in various sitting or reclining positions in small groups or alone scattered throughout the room.

The conversation stopped. They watched me warily as I took off my jacket. Some parents were in the room, standing in small groups of three or four. I turned to the kids. "Do you want your parents to be here while we talk?" Some sullen expressions returned my gaze, some sad. A few faces were mottled, eyes swollen from crying. "No," someone said quietly, and others indicated agreement.

"I am sorry," I told the parents. "You are going to have to leave." The parents nodded and quietly left the room. Two teachers remained. We began the meeting by setting ground rules. "Anyone can talk. No one must speak if they don't want to for any reason. No one is to judge anyone. Everyone is allowed to express what they think or know or feel without negative responses from anyone here."

"So, can you tell me what happened?" I indicated the kid closest to me on the right. He shook his head no. I asked the girl next to him, and she began slowly, reluctantly, to speak. "Henry went home that day.... He hung himself in the basement.... He's dead."

"Who told you?"

"My mom. She hung up the phone and started crying, and she told me."

"What were the words she used?"

"She said, 'Moira, I am sorry. Henry is dead.' I said, 'Henry? Which Henry?' And then she told me that it was Henry Newman, our classmate."

"Then what did you do?"

"I asked, 'How?' and she said he hung himself."

"And?"

"And I cried and went to Maya to tell her, and then we cried together."

Maya was sitting next to her, and she took up the narrative. "Yes, she came over, and when she told me, I thought she must be joking—a sick joke—it couldn't be true."

"And you?" I asked the next in the circle. And the discussion continued. It was very intense, some of the kids speaking, some preferring not to.

We spoke about the trauma of suicide, of who Henry was. Had anyone seen it coming? The guilt of survivors, the shock. Then in order to prepare them for what might be coming, I spoke to them about normal grief symptoms: difficulty in falling asleep, or wanting to sleep all the time; early morning awakenings; nightmares; eating a lot, or barely being able to swallow a mouthful; hallucinations of the dead classmate, either auditory or visual; guilt after so close a brush with death without having been able to prevent it. And more. At the end of the discussion, there were a few questions: "How long will we feel like this?" "How long will we remember him?"

Afterward, I took two chairs and put them in a corner of the room facing the corner so that anyone who had a question they didn't want to ask in front of the others could come and ask privately. They began to come, one at a time, to talk. The meeting lasted another two and a half hours. A lot of the questions were the same, and then one thirteen-year-old girl, Sadie, came to sit with me.

"I'm scared."

"What are you scared of?"

"I am a girl who really likes a lot of attention."

"And?"

"And I see that Henry is really the center of attention with everyone now." She looked down at her hands.

"And . . ."

"I am afraid that I might want to kill myself to be the center of attention."

There was a short silence.

"Is there life after death, Sadie?"

"Oh, yes."

"And can Henry see us now?"

"Yes, he can."

"So, he is enjoying all of the attention he is getting now?"

"Well, he didn't like attention so much, but he is probably enjoying it from there. Yes."

"Sadie, do you remember when another classmate of yours was killed in a car accident three years ago?"

"Yes."

"Did she get a lot of attention?"

"Oh, yes," she said enthusiastically. "We talked about her, and we cried all of the time. We made a memory book for her and did lots of stuff."

"Does anyone talk about her now, Sadie?" I asked quietly.

She sat in silence for a few moments. "Well, no. Not really. Maybe on her birthday or the anniversary of her death."

"Does she get as much attention now as, let's say, the least popular girl in your class?"

"Well, no, I don't think so."

"Sadie, all of the attention when someone dies calms down after only a few months. You will get much more attention if you stay alive."

She looked up intently and then wiped her face and smiled.

"Thank you. Oh, thank you so much."

One of the dangers of suicide, which is not relevant to other causes of death, is that it is infectious. This is illustrated with Sadie's response to Henry's death. Frequently in the wake of a suicide, we can see suicidal ideas with friends, relatives—even fans of a popular entertainment figure who commits suicide. This tendency must be identified early in order to prevent additional tragedies. As with any expressed suicidal thoughts, it is important not to ignore or try to brush off the rationale for a "copycat" suicide, but rather to try to address it inside the framework of the person who feels it. That was the source of this question to Sadie. Does Henry feel the attention he is getting, and how does he feel about it? The limited time span he will be receiving attention was used in this case as a deterrent to her "solution" of "copycat" suicide.

Because of the danger involved, the intervention could not be limited to those few sentences that Sadie and I exchanged. In keeping with the legal and moral requirement to report danger to others or oneself, the teacher needed to be alerted to keep an eye on her, and her parents needed to be alerted to watch for any unusual behavior. Sadie was informed that her teacher and parents would be alerted. In the event that there is no appropriate answer for Sadie, an immediate referral for professional help via psychological intervention would be necessary.

Where did the solution come from? The solution is usually embedded in the problem or the phrasing of the question. Generally speaking, questions or dilemmas about dying are practical and need to be addressed in a practical way. When someone is feeling like she is in danger, as Sadie did, she needs practical answers to serious questions. Very occasionally, one runs into a philosophical question that has the same impact as a practical one.

Following a trauma, because of the forbidden nature of talking about death, people are embarrassed to raise questions that they think might mark them as odd or different from others, or that might invite ridicule. For this reason, it is usually wise to provide the opportunity to ask questions privately. As one gathers more information from questions over the years, more of the answers can be included in the general debriefing or talk to the group to help them realize that normal feelings are indeed normal.

CONCLUSIONS

- *Following a suicide for any reason, survivors in the family and friends should be checked for suicidal ideas.*
- *Making a time and place for relatives or friends to voice their feelings and concerns, without being judged for the nature of the concern, is an important part of debriefing.*
- *Relating on a practical level to voiced concerns is an important part of prevention of additional tragedies following a suicide.*

REFERENCES

1. "The rate of suicide is twice as high in families of suicide victims as in comparison families. A family history of suicide predicted suicide independent of severe mental disorder. Whatever the mechanism for familial transmission of suicidal behavior may be, caution is justified in the aftermath of suicide. Supportive interventions may be indicated for the families of suicide victims" (B. Runeson & M. Asberg, "Family History of Suicide among Suicide Victims," *American Journal of Psychiatry* 160 [2003]: 1525–1526).

16

You Cannot Prepare

◠

Rehearsing Grief / Romanticizing Death

Following a three-day seminar titled "Dealing with Death," Ofira, a woman in her forties, came to me and said, "I have a problem I am embarrassed to discuss. In fact, I am afraid to talk about it at all. I have never told anyone before." She paused. "I am really afraid that one or all of my children will die. I live and breathe this fear. It is like a stone in my chest. Sometimes it even blocks my breathing. I feel the weight of it with me always. Even telling you now makes it more frightening for me." She looked down at her hands clenched together on the table where we were sitting at right angles. She looked up.

"Are your children in any real and present danger of death?" I asked. "Illness, extreme sports, army, drug or alcohol abuse, mental illness, depression, suicide attempts?"

"No, nothing at all. This fear has always been with me. Since they were very small, every day, all the years. What should I do? Can you help me? Am I normal?"

We sat in silence for a few moments.

"There are two possibilities, Ofira. Either none of your children will die in your lifetime. In this case, your time is totally wasted on trying to prepare yourself for an event that will never occur. The other possibility is that you are right, and one or more of your children will die while you are still alive. If that is the case, know that no amount of imagining or rehearsing for the death of a child will help you or prepare you for the impact of their death. The death of a child and the impact it carries with it is unimaginable. At the most, we picture ourselves being comforted or not, in the moment of death or at the graveyard. That is not grief. That is Hollywood.

"Grief over a child is not like other grief. There is really no way at all to immunize yourself emotionally against it. This means that if you are using the time you have with your children for this concern, know that this time that could be spent interacting with them is wasted. So in either case, it is a waste of time. Stop wasting your time."

Ofira stared at me for a full minute. "Thank you," she replied. "Thank you very much."

A week later, she sent an e-mail: "Life has changed since we spoke." She wrote, "I have been able to let it go. Thank you."

Although there are things we can do to prepare ourselves for an easier or cleaner grief period following a death, as illustrated in other stories in this book, there is no way to prepare for the individual impact of any given death. Death can have a different level of impact due to several specific variables.

One of these variables is related to the order in which deaths occur. The order of grandfather dying, then father, then son is usually easier from a grief standpoint than the son dying first, followed by father or grandfather. "Wrong-order death" is considered more difficult to bear than "right-order death." We expect death to occur in a certain sequence, from elder to younger, and when it does not occur in that way, we feel shaken and vulnerable. What can we trust anymore, if parents can bury their own child?

People who have experienced right-order death may believe that they understand what the impact of the death of a child (wrong-order death) would be. This is a mistaken assumption. The death of a child carries with it extra implications. For example, it is extremely common for the parent of a child who has died for any reason to feel guilt about the death. This guilt is attached to the parental imperative of protecting our children: "If my child has died, it must mean I have failed in my role of protector. I am therefore a failure as a parent and not an adequate shield for my remaining children."

To understand the futility of "rehearsal" for a death, we can look back in our lives at other significant events. Readers who are women and who have given birth to children, think back to the first live birth. You had probably tried to prepare for it, which may have included books, stories from friends and relatives, and perhaps classes in Lamaze or another form of assistance during birth. Think of how you thought the birth would be as opposed to how it in fact played out.

This analogy can apply to any life-changing event: marriage, raising children, changing jobs, or moving to another country, and so on. Our expectations and reality never match up one to one. Although there is value in preparing for events such as speeches, plays, tests, and so on, the degree of actual possible preparedness for the impact of the death and loss of a loved one is small.

> ## CONCLUSIONS
>
> - *Rehearsal does not prepare you for the impact of grief over a death, particularly the death of a child.*
> - *Imagination or rehearsing for a death that may or may not come in your lifetime uses a lot of energy that could be better spent on other things—for example, nurturing the cherished relationship itself.*

REFERENCES

1. "No one can ever fully prepare for grief even when they have nursed a loved one through a terminal illness" (M. W. Beck, "Sudden Loss Complicates Grief," www.centrahealth.com/news/digest/mar05/article2.aspx, accessed January 12, 2007).

2. "Some researchers report that anticipatory grief rarely occurs. They support this observation by noting that the periods of acceptance and recovery usually observed early in the grieving process are rarely found before the patient's actual death, no matter how early the forewarning. In addition, they note that grief implies that there has been a loss; to accept a loved one's death while he or she is still alive can leave the bereaved vulnerable to self-accusation for having partially abandoned the dying patient." . . . Although anticipatory grief may be therapeutic for families and other caregivers, there is concern that the dying person may experience too much grief, thus creating social withdrawal and detachment. Research indicates that widows usually remain involved with their dying husbands until the

time of death. This suggests that it was dysfunctional for the widows to have begun grieving in advance of their husbands' deaths. The widows could begin to mourn only after the actual death took place" ("Anticipatory Grief," from the Web page of the National Cancer Institute on Supportive Care, "Statement for Health Professionals: Loss, Grief, and Bereavement," www.meb .uni-bonn.de/cancer.gov/CDR0000062821.html#REF_23.2, accessed February 2, 2007).

3. "Death poses a threat and is an object of dread for many persons.... [It has been] found that 16.1% of the general population had a fear of death, 3.3% had an intense fear of death, and .5% had thanatophobia. Such fear may be secondary ... in some.... In others, the same fear may be primary. Death has many facets and threatens persons with loss of control or powerlessness, separation or alienation, loss of freedom or meaninglessness, as well as punishment" (R. Noyes Jr., S. Stuart, S. L. Longley, D. R. Langbehn, & R. L. Happel, "Hypochondriasis and Fear of Death," *Journal of Nervous and Mental Disease* 190 [2002]: 503–509).

17

I Can't Tell You

~

Getting Someone to Tell You Something

When she came to see me, she was very distressed over the death of the young girl she had been caring for. They had become very close during the past eighteen months. Now, two months after the death of her charge, Paula was finding it hard to cope. She didn't really feel she had the right to mourn because she wasn't a family member. But since the death, her life had lost meaning and direction.

At one point in our conversation, I asked Paula if she had ever thought of harming herself.

"Yes, I think about it all the time."

"Do you have a plan?"

She described an easily accomplished, well-thought-out plan to kill herself, and she had taken care to acquire the means to do it.

"When do you plan to carry this out?"

"Maybe later today, maybe tomorrow . . ."

"You realize that I can't let you leave here without making sure you are safe. Who would you like me to call—police, hospital, family physician?"

She gave me a number, and I called her family physician and made the necessary arrangements.

Paula was admitted to a mental hospital for suicidal clinical depression. From time to time she would call, and we would talk for five or ten minutes on the phone. After a time, she was released and continued to attend day programs at the hospital.

A few months after that she called. "I really need to meet with you."

"Paula, you have a psychologist and a psychiatrist. You would not be doing yourself a favor to be getting counseling also from me. Everyone works in their own way, and it will become too confusing."

A day later, she called again. "I really need just one meeting with you. I have arranged everything. It is really important, please."

"Okay, I will be in your village tomorrow, and we can meet."

The next day in her home, she made coffee, and we sat down. I was on a couch and she on a comfortable chair at right angles to the couch.

"So, Paula, why did you want to meet?"

"Just to talk."

"What would you like to talk about?"

"We're getting a lot of rain this year. It's good."

"Yes . . . is there anything else?"

"Not really . . . "

"You sounded pretty urgent on the phone. What was it you wanted to talk to me about at that time?"

"Oh, nothing."

"Okay. Are you still thinking about killing yourself?"

"Yes."

"Still the same method?"

"Yes."

"I have a very hard question to ask you." In reality, I had no such question, but I watched her rearrange her seating and steel herself.

"What is the question?"

"Do you love your son?" (She had a four-year-old son, an only child.)

"Oh, yes—I guess so. I thought you were going to ask something much harder."

"What did you think I was going to ask?"

"I can't tell you."

"Okay. Tell me, Paula, are you thinking of murdering your son and then committing suicide?"

She looked startled, and then blurted: "Yes!"

"Why?"

"Because every time I tell someone I don't want to live or I want to commit suicide, people tell me, 'But think of your child.' So I am thinking of him."

"Did you tell your psychologist that this is your plan?"

"I tried, but he said, 'You just want to manipulate us into taking you back to the hospital.'"

"Can you please give me his phone number?"

She did, and I went into another room to make the call to Paula's psychologist and explained the situation.

"She is just using manipulation to get back into the hospital," he said.

"Listen very carefully. I am not a psychologist or a psychiatrist, but I know very well that there is no way you can know if a suicide or murder threat is serious or not. She has the idea, she has the means; you cannot ignore this situation."

"She is just using an empty threat."

"All right. So now you will hear a threat that is not empty. If you do not immediately hospitalize this woman for being a danger to herself and her child, you will never counsel in this country again."

She was hospitalized within hours.

Paula weathered the crisis, and she still gets in touch with me from time to time.

Many people who commit suicide see physicians within three months prior to the act. Most, as Paula did, will answer directly to a direct question about the intent to commit suicide.

Suicide, however, is a taboo subject. Many people (even counselors and medical personnel) are afraid that by asking, they may actually be giving the person the idea to use the suicide option. Yet research has shown that this is actually not true.

Most people who are grieving have at least thought of suicide or not being alive in passing. Answers to a direct question will vary:

1. "Yes, but it's not for me."
2. "Yes, but it's against my religion."
3. "I could never do that to my loved ones."
4. "I haven't the courage or strength to do it."
5. "Yes, I have saved up hundreds of pills, but I want to wait till my daughter gets married"

(*When will that be?*) "I have no idea when; she hasn't met the right man yet."

Or, they may describe a well-planned and available time, means, and/or place, as in Paula's case.

This is a line of questioning many people, both professionals and laypeople, don't like to initiate. It's born of an assumption that talking about suicide will make a precarious situation more dangerous. If someone brings up the fact that they are considering suicide, we don't want to listen or to repeat to anyone else the possibility. But because we have no sure way of knowing whether or not a suicide plan is likely to be carried out, we have to take all such expressions at face value. It is important to ascertain the seriousness of the threat or to make sure the individual sees someone who can make this assessment.

One way to assess the seriousness is to explore the speaker's personal history. In Paula's case, her personal history included suicidal depression. An additional determining factor is whether or not the speaker has a viable plan to carry out the threat. For one individual, this might be an acquired weapon, whether pills or a gun; for another, it can be a place and a time.

Just because someone contemplating suicide has a support system in place does not mean the support system is functioning properly. So it is important to ask. Paula had a support system in place in a mental health framework. She had advisers, counselors, and group support. Somehow it was not functioning to her satisfaction, and she insisted on looking for help outside this support system.

If a grieving person begins to elaborate on a threat and then hides the details or, like Paula, hints that they are in a crisis and then will not explain, it is possible to "shock" the vital information out of them by the "wild-guess method."

As Clifton K. Meador, M.D., advises in his *Little Book of Doctors' Rules* (Philadelphia: Hanley & Belfus, 1992), if a patient is afraid to tell you some piece of information, guess the most outrageous, horrible thing you can think of. You will get one of the following results: (1) You will be correct and appear to be clairvoyant. (2) Your suggestion will sound so horrible that whatever they were going to say will seem less horrible by comparison, and then they can tell you the (relatively) tame truth.

CONCLUSIONS

- *Do not be afraid to ask mourners if they are thinking of hurting themselves.*
- *Do not ignore suicidal intentions but assess how serious they are or inform someone who can.*
- *Knowing there is a support system in place does not necessarily mean it is functioning properly.*

REFERENCES

1. "Warning signs of suicide are usually evident and family members of those who have committed suicide may not be aware of these signs. . . . Family members may not be aware of suicide warning signs in their suicidal relatives" (M. G. Mac-Donald, "Suicide-Intervention Trainees' Perceptions of Awareness for Warning Signs of Suicide," *Psychological Reports* 85 [1999]: 1195–1198).

2. "Bereavement support is an integral part of palliative care. Grieving after loss is a normal process; however, some grief reactions become complicated and may seriously compromise the health of an individual. Routine bereavement care helps identify people at risk of complicated grieving. The burden of grief can last for years, sometimes indefinitely. People caring for the bereaved need to pay special attention to cultural differences, the burden of caring for dying children, and the special support needs of bereaved children and adolescents. Excellent resources to assist in grief management, including the expertise of palliative care teams, are readily available" (I. Maddocks, "Grief and Bereavement," *Medical Journal of Australia* 179, 6 Suppl. [2003]: S6–7).

18

Letting Go

TAKING CHANCES
WITH COMMUNICATION

AN OLDER MAN, Eli, wasted because of his disease, sat in a large brown chair in a clean, comfortable home. He was covered with a wool blanket, despite the fact that the house was warm. His wife, Karen, was sitting on a low chair at his right side. She was smiling and welcoming. He was not.

She invited me to sit, but before I could take the proffered seat, Eli began to shout at me. "You have to tell me how to end all this!"

"Excuse me?"

He began again. "You must help me to end all of this." He gestured, palm inward toward his body with disgust.

"Sorry, I cannot help you end your life."

Again, louder, angrier: "You have to help me finish this!"

"Tell me why I have to help you finish this." I was still standing.

Karen was trying to calm him down with "shh" noises and saying, "Don't excite yourself, Eli."

"This body is falling apart! I am losing all semblance of humanity! I am a burden to everyone, especially myself! I can't take it anymore! I am dying! You must do it!"

"I am sorry, Eli. I cannot help you to end your life."

"Do you know how to end my life?"

"Yes. But I won't help you end your life."

He began screaming. "Don't you understand?! I am dying! I have a problem!"

I bent over and leaned toward him and looked directly at him, speaking in a quiet voice. "Yes. You have a problem. But your problem is temporary. You are dying."

There was silence in the room for about two minutes.

Eli spoke again, this time in a normal voice. "Then why did you come?"

"To help you decide what you want to do with the time you have left."

There was another moment of silence, and then Eli beckoned to a chair near him. "Please sit down."

We spoke for about an hour, until Eli was too tired to continue. We spoke of making peace with himself and with those around him. He told me about his past: whom he felt he treated fairly and whom he did not; who he felt treated him badly and why. We spoke about forgiveness and the price of unforgiveness; about expressing his feelings and dealing with them directly, rather than continuing to simmer them over a low fire. We spoke of death and fears and his view of what comes after death. He told me about his difficulties with perfectionism and his relationship with his children in light of his need for control.

He left to go to sleep, and I spoke for another hour with Karen. Karen said that her life with Eli had been very hard. Eli was a controlling man, who had been married prior to his marriage to Karen. His first wife had had an affair with his best friend. Karen, who was many years Eli's junior, had been forced to bear the brunt of that betrayal. Eli had needed to know where she was every moment of every day, for over eighteen years. Despite his extreme jealousy, Karen had started a cottage industry, which had become a very successful international business over the years.

We met again the following week. Then Eli's illness worsened; he was hospitalized and died shortly thereafter. A month later, after the thirty-day memorial of Eli's death, Karen came to see me. She related to me that Eli had undergone a transformation in the last six weeks of his life. I asked her what she thought the trigger for the transformation could have been.

She said, "It was the first meeting with you."

"What was the nature of this transformation?"

"Before, we used to have to walk on eggs. He could explode at any wrong word, and we never knew which words were wrong. Then he changed. He became softer, more pliable. He became more quiet and thoughtful . . . and then he wanted to have serious talks with all those he was close to.

"They were emotional talks, but not filled with anger and manipulation, as was the norm in our family. It was different— he was reviewing his life with each of us. He spoke about pain he had felt and pain he had caused. Apologizing . . . Can you believe it—Eli apologizing?!

"Every conversation drained out a little more anger or bitterness. He began to really listen to our son, and to me. And he became more peaceful as he was able to resolve every relationship.

He made peace with our son. He made peace with his business associates, with neighbors, and friends—and with himself. It was amazing. He lost his anger. He became peaceful and relaxed.

"The day before he died, we were in the hallway of the hospital. He was lying on a gurney, and I was standing beside him. Then he turned to me and said, 'Karen, take off your wedding ring and give it to me.' I did so. He took off his own wedding ring, looked at them both, put them together in his hand, then reached over and put them both in my pocket. He said to me, 'Karen, you are released. Whenever you are ready for the second chapter of your life [a new partner], feel free to pursue it. If it is in three days, three weeks, three months, or three years. I release you from any obligation to me.'"

Why was Eli so furious? What was really going on? Eli was furious because no one was really communicating with him, and he couldn't communicate with them either. However, anger was a long-standing problem with Eli. It didn't begin with his disease.

It must be recognized that someone in a life-threatening situation may communicate in odd, bizarre, or (as in Eli's case) desperate ways. This is natural, although not everyone will choose the communication style that Eli used.

When I first met Eli, the overwhelming message from him was anger and rage. It was not just that he spoke directly, rather than through symbolism (as the dying person did in chapter 4, "The Black Place"). It was also apparent in his face: jaw thrust forward, eyes flashing, eyebrows drawn together. His voice was demanding, loud, aggressive, with deep breathing.

In addition to the verbal and body language he was using, his wife Karen was trying to calm him down, and he was ignoring her completely. So it was apparent that trying to pacify Eli would be ineffective.

When someone shouts it usually means they feel they are not being heard. Eli was telling me how to speak to him. Repeating what he had said back to him was the only way to assure him that I indeed had heard him. He was then able to speak in a normal tone.

Sometimes we need to take a direct approach, yet in another situation it might be highly inappropriate. Communication must be tailored to the individual, or we risk causing them to feel that we don't hear them, and then they won't hear us.

There is usually more than one way to communicate in any given situation. While one way may be more effective, a slightly less effective way can also yield results, albeit more slowly. It is important to carefully observe the person who is speaking, taking into account our own experience and normal communication style. If we pay close attention, we can get to the general style that will work in a particular case. According to the person's responses, we can perceive when we are closer to, or further from, a style that is comfortable for him.

CONCLUSIONS

- *Someone who is suffering and feeling threatened by impending destruction may indicate this by communicating in strange or aggressive ways.*
- *The narrative, both verbal and nonverbal (body language), is the story. The person you are communicating with will show you the best way to reach him.*
- *Pay attention to the environment, including any other communication going on and its effectiveness or lack of effectiveness.*
- *Several ways of communicating will work to varying degrees with a given individual. It is usually enough to approach the general style and then move as close to it as our own style will allow.*

REFERENCES

1. "When we see a bodily expression of emotion, we immediately know what specific action is associated with a particular emotion, leaving little need for interpretation of the signal, as is the case for facial expressions. Research on emotional body language is rapidly emerging as a new field in cognitive and affective neuroscience. This article reviews how whole-body signals are automatically perceived and understood, and their role in emotional communication and decision-making" (B. de Gelder, "Towards the Neurobiology of Emotional Body Language," *Nature Reviews Neuroscience* 7 [2006]: 242–249).

2. "When face and body convey conflicting emotional information, judgment of facial expression is hampered and becomes

biased toward the emotion expressed by the body" (H. K. Meeren, C. C. van Heijnsbergen, & B. de Gelder, "Rapid Perceptual Integration of Facial Expression and Emotional Body Language," *Proceedings of the National Academy of Sciences of the United States of America* 102 [2005]: 16518–16523).

3. "We all know that what we don't say can be as important as what we do say. In this fascinating piece of research Lesley Mason describes how she was able to relate the non-verbal communication of interview candidates to the outcome of the interview" (L. Mason, "Body Language—Non-verbal Cues," *British Journal of Perioperative Nursing* 10 [2000]: 512–518).

19

What Is the Gain?

～

COST VERSUS BENEFIT

IT HAD BEEN MONTHS SINCE Shai's disease first showed itself. This disease would kill this small boy. By the lost look of his father, Benjamin, it appeared that it might kill him too.

This illness was vicious, taking any small gains Shai had managed in his four years of life and slowly reversing them, until this child who had run and played with all his friends was now bedridden. He had only power to slightly move the ends of his fingers. He couldn't even breathe unassisted. It was as if all his muscles had melted away. His life would probably be over within the year. In the meantime, the struggle was with the pain and with his father's hopelessness. Shai somehow managed to enjoy every small attention. Could it be that he didn't remember that less than half a year ago, he had been running with his friends?

Benjamin and I met, as we did weekly, to talk about setbacks, frustrations, and how to plan your life, your week, your day . . . or only your hour, when your only child was living in the deep shadow of death.

After about twenty minutes the words ran out, as often happened in these meetings. There was not always a way to mold pain into syllables. We sat in silence for a while. Then Benjamin turned and looked at me without speaking.

"Benjamin," I began, "What have you gained from Shai's illness?"

"What?!" he whispered hoarsely. "What could I have possibly gained?"

I waited a moment before continuing. "Benjamin, for everything in life—everything—there is a price and a possibility of profit. Everything."

"I don't understand."

"Every situation, however horrible, carries with it a possibility of a gift, a gain, a benefit. The price and the benefit are not usually equal. Sometimes, as with Shai, the price is unspeakable and the gain may be small. Sometimes, the price is small and the gain large or any combination in between.

"The difference between the price and the benefit is that the price is fixed. You cannot change it. You cannot avoid it. The benefit is optional. You usually have to look hard just to find it. It is frequently hard to agree to take the gain because it seems somehow profane to benefit from, for example, Shai's pain or illness."

He continued to look at me silently, waiting for me to continue.

"There is always the possibility of a gain. It is an option—you can take it or leave it. Whichever you choose, it doesn't affect the price in any way."

"So what should I do?" Benjamin asked helplessly.

"First look for the benefit. Then decide."

"What possible benefit could there be?"

"It could be anything. Changes you have had to make to accommodate your son's illness—changes that could be good."

He thought for a few moments.

"All my life, I've been shy, afraid, really, of any confrontation. I made sure I was always in the background, or I would agree with everyone. Anything to avoid confrontation." He looked down at the floor for a moment and then looked up.

"And?"

He paused. "I have had to fight with everyone. It took a long time to figure out what was happening to Shai. I knew something was wrong, but everyone insisted I was being hysterical. I insisted on a second opinion, then a third opinion. I brought him to the best doctors in the country, insisted on medical coverage. I had to fight for him. I learned to fight! I learned to fight. " He began to cry. "I learned to fight . . . " he murmured.

I waited until Benjamin's tears subsided and his eyes met mine.

"Benjamin," I said, "This is a gift from Shai. Don't lose it."

CONCLUSIONS

- *With every situation comes a price and the possibility of a benefit.*
- *The price is fixed, and the benefit is optional.*
- *If you are already paying the price, it is wise to take the benefit.*
- *Whether you take or leave the benefit, the price remains the same.*

REFERENCES

1. "Nothing in the whole world is meaningless, suffering least of all" (Oscar Wilde, *De Profundis*).

2. "There is also purpose in that life which is almost barren of both creation and enjoyment and which admits of but one possibility of high moral behavior: namely, in man's attitude to his existence, and existence restricted by external forces. . . . Without suffering and death human life cannot be complete" (V. E. Frankl, *Man's Search for Meaning: An Introduction to Logotherapy*, trans. I. Lasch [1946; reprint, New York: Washington Square Press, 1963], p. 106; "He who has a why to live for can bear with almost any how" (Friedrich Nietzsche, quoted in ibid., p. 121).

20

Body Language

◦——

THE CLARITY OF AFFECTIVE
COMMUNICATION

SAFRA WAS A PSYCHOLOGIST who came for supervision. Safra had chosen to work with support groups of cancer victims, along with other people who had sustained a particularly tough trauma. She told me that she needed to be less emotionally involved with her clients and their pain.

I asked her to describe a typical meeting with the group of cancer victims. She talked of sitting in a group as one of its members described some aspect of her battle with disease. Safra added, "She said this, and my stomach turned over . . . " And as she spoke, she clutched at her lower stomach, her body jerked a bit forward, and her face reflected agonizing pain. She then related another event in the group, using the same terminology and the same body language. And then—for the third time— she described a different exchange in the group, using the same gestures.

By this time, I was paying close attention to all details of her body language, almost to the exclusion of her verbal message. She stopped speaking and looked at me expectantly.

"I have been working in this field for many years."

She replied, "I know—that's why I wanted to come to you."

Leaning forward intently, speaking slowly and deliberately, I said: "In all the years I have been working with the sick, the bereaved, and the dying, my stomach has never turned over from a counselee's story."

She looked shocked, then said tentatively, "I thought everybody felt the same way I do when they are counseling."

"No. Now, I want you to tell me your own personal story about your cancer in the area of your lower stomach."

She stared at me, stunned. "Who told you?"

"Your body language did, when you spoke about the group meeting."

"Oh." She paused. "I will tell you the story, but why is it so important?"

"If you keep on running from your own story of cancer, you will continue to be too wounded by it to help with anyone else's battle without repercussions to yourself."

In the realm of communication, body language (also called "affective communication") plays a significant role. In our encounters with other individuals, it is wise to pay attention not only to their verbal communication but also to their body language. Body language will sometimes reveal things that are not clear from the words, as with Safra.

In every meeting that we have with another individual, for any purpose, there are two worlds colliding: our own and that of the other person. Sometimes the collision is mild, no more than a gentle nudge. Other times the two cultures, personalities, or life histories may clash powerfully. During such a collision, many things can erupt, whether or not they are expressed. Sometimes, as in Safra's case, the impact can open old wounds; occasionally, it can open new ones—or none at all, despite the force of the collision.

One of the realities to keep in mind is that everyone has a history and a culture. In addition, each person has been through his or her own "stuff," ordeals that may have involved loss, pain, sorrow, trauma—or a combination of all of them. It is safe to assume that everyone is carrying something.

The caretaker type of individual is particularly prone to forget about her or his own "baggage." This refers not only to those who make a living from counseling and caretaking roles, but also those who frequently find themselves taking on such roles for others. Caretakers need to keep in mind that they also have needs, history, and culture; and if they don't take care of themselves, they will find it quite difficult to care for others in the long term. This advice is similar to the routine instruction given by flight attendants before an airplane takes off: in case of emergency, first apply the oxygen mask to your own face, and then assist children or dependents with putting on theirs.

Taking care of oneself can be done in many ways. Many times we think that this can be accomplished on our own, relying on our personal resources and having faith in our potential. In my experience, self-reliance does not provide enough support to the caretaker for the long term. It is important to know how to ask for and receive help outside ourselves. Sometimes it is necessary to seek professional help, as Safra did, or a colleague's assistance. Sometimes the help involves an informal support system, such as friends who know how to listen. Sometimes it comes through faith in G-d and a support system involving prayer. Or it could be any combination of these things.

CONCLUSIONS

- *Paying attention to body language can give you an invaluable "window" into what the other person is really communicating.*
- *Everyone is carrying "baggage"; no one comes empty-handed to an encounter with another individual.*
- *You have to take care of yourself before (and while) dealing with those under your care, or you may become incapable of helping them.*

REFERENCES

1. "Whenever they can, individual physicians should be attentive to their practices and modify their work environment to reduce stressors so as to enhance their wellness. Coping mechanisms such as stress management, family support, recreation, hobbies or participation in support groups are among possible resources that may help . . . prevent fatigue, stress or burn out" (S. Taub, K. Morin, M. S. Goldrich, P. Ray, R. Benjamin, & Council on Ethical and Judicial Affairs of the American Medical Association, "Physician Health and Wellness," *Occupational Medicine* 56 [March 2006]: 77–82).

2. "Physicians use a variety of approaches to promote their own well-being, which sort themselves into 5 main categories and appear to correlate with improved levels of psychological well-

being among users . . . 'relationships,' 'religion or spirituality,' 'self-care,' 'work,' and 'approaches to life.' . . . The last type . . . was significantly associated with increased psychological well-being" (E. L. Weiner, G. R. Swain, B. Wolf, & M. Gottlieb, "A Qualitative Study of Physicians' Own Wellness-Promotion Practices," *Western Journal of Medicine* 174 [2001]: 19–23).

21

Harps in Heaven, Accordions in Hell

CHANGING PERCEPTIONS

SIX CHILDREN WERE SITTING on small chairs around a large table in the art room of the children's hospital. They were between the ages of six and nine years.

They all had some things in common. They were all bereaved of a sibling who had died from a long illness. They all had had to live with the sick sibling at the center of their family's focus for a long time. And now, even when the sick child was no longer alive, it was apparent to all of them that he or she still remained at the center of their grieving family's focus. These children had not only to deal with their own grief and loss, but also with their parents' inability to invest in the remaining children.

In the past weeks, the children had done many art projects, speaking more freely when their hands were busy than they did in one-to-one conversation. All of the projects were designed to assist them with their grief, whether for their sibling, their parents, or themselves.

Jenna, a seven-year-old girl from a religious home, was smearing clay with her fingers on construction paper and speaking aloud to no one in particular. She frequently fought with other children in the group, occasionally even storming off and slamming the door, only to reappear a few minutes later and continue her project, tears still smudged on her cheeks.

"My mother is sinning. She is a terrible mother," Jenna announced without looking up.

"Why is she a terrible mother?" I asked moving quietly to her side.

"She cries all the time. She never stops, and she is always crying over Saul."

"Why does this make her a terrible mother?"

"The rabbi, when he came to our home during Shiva [the formal mourning period], he told us."

"What did he tell you?"

"He told us not to cry for Saul. He told us if we cry, then Saul will be punished in heaven." She added some clay to her picture, got up and looked at it from a standing position, sat down satisfied and reached for a marker.

"What kind of punishment did the rabbi talk about for Saul?"

"He said Saul will not be allowed to attend Bible lessons up there if we cry for him. Mom always cries for him, so he cannot go. She is a terrible mother. She is sinning." She hummed for a bit, added another smear of colored clay, and then got up to drink some juice.

Here was an unusual dilemma. In the world of the Jewish religious child, the rabbi is the final authority. As a counselor, there was no challenging a rabbi's authority to a religious child.

There was no question about the rabbi's sincerity. If Jenna had understood him correctly, then perhaps he had thought he would help the family recover by stopping their tears. But regardless of what he had actually said, this child and her relationship with her mother were suffering, and would continue to do so, because of either what he had said or how Jenna had interpreted his words. How could this be stopped?

After drinking her juice, Jenna had seated herself in the Lego corner. I sat down on the floor near her.

"Jenna, what is heaven like?"

She attached a few more Lego blocks to the thing she had begun making. She didn't look up as she began to describe a child's heaven. She described something that sounded more or less like Disneyland plus Bible lessons.

"Wow! Sounds pretty amazing. So Saul is up there?"

"Yep," she said confidently, adding another Lego to her block.

"So . . . what? Your mom is crying that Saul is in such a great place?" She looked at me for the first time in a while.

"Umm . . ."

"Do you think your mom would cry over Saul being in a place like that?"

She continued to look at me. "No . . . I don't think so . . ."

"So, maybe . . . maybe she isn't crying for Saul."

She watched me curiously.

"Maybe she's crying for herself because she misses him."

"Maybe," she said uncertainly.

"Oh," I said with surprise. "Well, then, that means that Saul can go into Bible lessons."

"He can?" she asked.

"Well, yeah, because your mom is crying for herself, not for him."

"Oh, yeah!" she replied happily.

"And you can cry when you miss him too, because it's you crying for you, not for Saul."

She smiled. "So, maybe my mom is not sinning?"

"I think you are right about that, Jenna."

Frequently when communicating with children, misunderstandings occur. We do know that Jenna *thought* the rabbi had said that her brother would be punished because of her mother's tears. This, then, was reality for Jenna. This, then, is the material that we have to work with.

There is usually more than one way to change someone's perception of a situation. One strategy is a direct confrontation. In a direct confrontation, we would force the child to choose sides, when he or she is not necessarily equipped or willing to do so. In this case, we would be taking a chance regarding on whose authority the child prefers to depend. Another strategy is to try to convince the child that she heard incorrectly. This is based on an assumption that we have no direct information to confirm or deny. It is not advisable to try changing anyone's perception (child or adult) with an uninformed assertion that may later collapse under the weight of reality. Once your credibility is called into question by such a mistake, it is very difficult to regain trust.

A third way to change a perception is to intentionally avoid conflict or direct confrontation by reinterpreting the information in a way that is less destructive to the child. In Jenna's case, this was an effective way of dealing with the conflict between her mother and herself. In this method, creative problem solving can be used. This doesn't have to be an innate talent; it can be learned. One way to cultivate this skill is to understand that there is always more than one way to look at any given situation, and there is always more than one way to solve a problem.

CONCLUSIONS

- *Reality is subjective, or seen through the eyes of personal experience, history, and culture. Therefore, in a secondhand report, we can never be sure of the actual intent or words used in the encounter. We must work instead with the perception of the mourner.*
- *If the understanding is destructive, either for the individual or for an individual's relationship with a significant other, it is wise to look for a way to make the understanding or perception more constructive.*
- *Several strategies are available to change someone's destructive perception of a situation, and care must be taken to choose a strategy that is likely to work with that individual.*

REFERENCES

1. "The prevalent approach to understanding of and clinical intervention in the process of mourning employs a model based on stages of bereavement. This paper suggests a theoretical conception that is not tied to a fixed order of emotional states. Two

dimensions—closeness of relationship and mourner's perception of preventability of the death—are identified as prime predictors of the intensity and duration of bereavement" (L. A. Bugen, "Human Grief: A Model for Prediction and Intervention," *American Journal of Orthopsychiatry* 47 [1977]: 196–206).

2. "The grief process is influenced by personal, cultural, and societal expectations and experiences, as well as the mourner's perception of the loss" (N. A. Carrington & J. F. Bogetz, "Normal Grief and Bereavement: Letters from Home," *Journal of Palliative Care Medicine* 7 [2004]: 309–323).

22

Waiting to Die

∽

THE TIMING OF DEATH

RUTH, THE MOTHER in the family, had called earlier that week. "My son is dying. The nurse in the hospital advised me to meet with you."

"Okay. When would you like to meet?"

"Well, I don't know. What do you charge?" I told her. "And what do I get for this money?"

"We sit and talk. You talk a little, I talk a little."

"And this is supposed to help?"

"I am told that it does."

"Okay. So let's meet." We set a time.

Now, we were sitting at a large round table in the family home, just the ten of us, two parents, seven adult children, and myself. One family member was not present. The eldest son, Jack, was hospitalized and dying.

Jack's story was a story of repeated remissions of cancer interspersed with active periods of the disease since he was eight
years old. He was now thirty-seven.

Everyone was active in the telling of the story, interrupting
and correcting one another, crying now and then. Everyone
except the father, Hershel, who sat with his back toward the
family, slumped as if a great weight was on his shoulders.

After they finished speaking, we began to talk about saying
goodbye. One of the daughters protested, "But if we all go one
by one to say goodbye, he's going to think he's dying!"

"Wait a minute—he's not dying? But you said he was."

"No, I mean he's dying, but if we do that he'll know he's
dying."

"Tell me. Does he have any brain damage?"

"No. He's very smart. Why would you say something like
that?"

"Well, because dying people usually know when they are
dying, at least on some level. Jack is in a cancer ward. He sees
others dying. He is losing function after function. You told me
Jack has been giving his possessions away and is asking to see
certain people 'one more time' that he hasn't seen in a while.
Jack knows he's dying. He's pretending everything is okay,
because that's what you are doing. He is protecting you. Give
Jack a chance not to be alone. He'll probably take it."

At the close of this meeting, Hershel remained slumped forward and uncommunicative.

About two months later, Ruth asked me to come again. In
the interim, Jack had died, been buried, and the thirtieth day
(a traditional time of visiting the graveyard) had passed since his
demise. The door to the family home was opened by Hershel,

who greeted me warmly with a two-handed handclasp and an arm around my shoulders ushering me in.

Everyone was waiting inside. Hershel seated me and said, "I must tell you what happened with Jack."

"Please do."

"We went to the hospital. All of his siblings made their farewells to him as you suggested, dealing with unfinished business where necessary. There were a lot of tears, but you know what? Jack was happy. He lost the haunted look in his eyes, and they were all just together. Yes, that's the word—'together.' Ruth also spoke to him at great length, and you could see how close they were. Only I was alone on the outside. Everyone was telling me I had to talk to Jack, but I couldn't. It was horrible. And then he lost consciousness. I felt like I would die with him . . . my son, my son."

Hershel rubbed his eyes with his knuckles.

"Then I remembered that you said that he might be able to hear me even if he were unconscious. I walked into his room. I walked back out. I walked in again and then out, three or four times. Finally, I sat down next to his bed, took his hand, and began to talk to him. I told him everything—how I loved him, how my dreams were crushed with his illness, how guilty I felt, and a lot of other things. Then I said goodbye to my son, whom I loved."

He stopped and bowed his head, and a few moments later raised his eyes to meet mine again.

"What happened?" I asked gently.

"As soon as I finished, he let out a long breath and died." Hershel's eyes were shining. "He was at peace," he said.

"He waited for you, Hershel."

"Yes."

"And moreover, he chose to die with your voice in his ears. This is a gift. Do not forget it."

"I won't," he replied.

Hershel's reaction to his son's illness and to professional intervention was not unusual. Many times we see this response with both adults and children. During a family counseling session, there may be one or more children off to the side, playing, apparently a thousand miles away from what is taking place in the room. Don't be deceived. Those who are in the room can hear everything, even if it is not apparent. People don't have to interact with us in order to hear us. We cannot always know what is going on according to the surface response or lack of it.

We are also familiar with the opposite effect: that of a person you are talking to who appears to be listening and is, in fact, not hearing you at all. This, again, is not a rare occurrence and is sometimes difficult to identify.

An additional reason for a family meeting that includes all members, regardless of active participation levels, is to prevent them from feeling left out or feeling that something is being hidden from them.

Many times, in the case of terminal illness, the dying person chooses their moment of death, within reasonable physical limitations. This moment of death frequently coincides with a final goodbye from a close family member or friend, even while the dying person is unconscious. The moment of death also sometimes coincides with a brief absence from the room of the dying person by someone who adamantly refuses to let them "give up" or who tells the unconscious person repeatedly to "hang on."

CONCLUSIONS

- *People don't have to interact with you to hear you. We cannot always tell by the outside reaction what is going on inside.*
- *People sometimes hear when unconscious.*
- *People who are dying of disease usually know it. Sometimes they choose the time to die, waiting for the release of final goodbyes, or waiting for a moment when relatives who are refusing to say goodbye have left the room.*

REFERENCES

1. "The article brings some evidence to support the idea that unconscious people appear to hear, or at least, their brains react to speech almost like a conscious person's. Whether they can interpret these sounds is not known" (D. Steinberg, "Revelations from the Unconscious—Can Vegetative and Minimally Conscious States Expose the Cerebral Substrates of Awareness?" *Scientist* 19 [2005]: 17; available online at www.the-scientist.com/article/display/15705/, accessed February 9, 2007).

2. "Comatose patients may, however, hear; many have normal brain-stem auditory evoked responses and normal physiologic responses to auditory stimuli. Not talking to comatose patients may promote the notion that they are dead or nearly dead; not talking may become a self-fulfilling prophecy, influencing physicians to inappropriately withhold or withdraw therapy. Because comatose patients are especially vulnerable, and because some comatose patients may recover, physicians should consider talking to these patients. Our analysis suggests that families,

medical students, and house staff would benefit from the humane example modeled by those clinicians who care for and talk to all patients" (J. La Puma, D. L. Schiedermayer, A. E. Gulyas, & M. Siegler, "Talking to Comatose Patients," *Archives of Neurology* 45 [1988]: 20–22).

23

Where Did You Get My Number?

∽

IDENTIFYING THE BEREAVED

WHILE I WAS DRIVING HOME from a lecture, my mobile phone rang.

"Hello?"

"Hello," an agitated voice responded. "You have to help me. My son has become crazy. He has lost it completely."

"Excuse me?"

"My son has lost his mind, and I don't know what to do!"

"Where did you get my number?"

"Jeanie, a friend, gave it to me a long time ago."

"I am not a psychologist or a psychiatrist."

"Yes, I know," she replied impatiently.

"I don't think you have the right phone number."

"I do."

"There may be some mistake."

"There is no mistake. You are the one I need to talk to."

"Okay . . . and what is going on?"

"My son has lost his mind."

"How old is he?"

"Eight."

"And what do you see that makes you say he has lost his mind?"

"He is screaming and tearing at his hair and scratching himself and throwing things around and breaking things."

"And how long has he been this way?"

"Since he woke up this morning."

I looked at the clock in the car. It was 11:22 in the morning. "What time did he wake up?"

"Around 9:30."

"So, he's been this way for about two hours?"

"Yes, yes, you have to help me."

"When he woke at 9:30, did he say anything about a nightmare?"

"No, he woke normally and a few minutes later began screaming and running around the house and breaking things."

"What happened in those few minutes between when he woke up and when he started screaming?"

"His father died."

My car suddenly swerved to the right. I pulled over to the side of the road.

"Excuse me. Could you repeat what you just said?"

"His father died at home a few minutes after he woke up."

"Is his father, by any chance, your husband?"

"Yes," she replied in a shaky voice.

If someone insists on talking to you, even if you think you are not the right person for the job, as in this story, listen and try to find out why they think you are. It may be that you are the right addressee, but they are unable to express why at this particular time. Clarification may require careful questioning.

It is not always obvious who the person needing the help is. It can be that the "identified patient" or the person identified as having problems is simply the "family thermometer"—the one through whom the family stress is expressed in a more obvious way than with other family members.

After a parental death, the surviving parent is trying to cope with many different tasks and conflicting emotions, and it can be hard for such parents to let their guard down enough to realize that they need help. "After all," the survivor may feel, "everyone is depending on me now. There is no one else to take care of the house, the kids, and the funeral arrangements, and now I'm the only wage earner." Ascertaining who needs help can be tricky.

This was also the case in this family. This may be because the parent is trying to control her own emotions and, in order to do so, has to repress them. It may be, in the case of men, that the masculine expectation of coping with trauma for him does not include tears or hysteria, or even lack of control. Perhaps the person is numbed by what happened and can only see the children and concerns about them and can't address personal needs at all.

If we refuse a person in this state, we may miss an important opportunity to support or assist someone in need. Again, as in other stories, it is important to recognize the necessity to listen carefully to the person who is speaking to you.

CONCLUSIONS

- *It is not always obvious who the needy person is. Careful questioning will usually reveal the facts.*
- *When someone is insistent that you are the person they need to speak to, it is important to find out why.*
- *Listen carefully to all that is said—every word is important.*

REFERENCES

1. "[This] resulted in his idea of the 'hidden patient'—caregivers who are vulnerable as a result of attending to family members with chronic and long-term illnesses. . . . Physicians who recognize the emotional and social aspects . . . will not only promote the health of the individual patient but also the wellbeing of their carers. . . . Hidden patients have various stress-related illnesses . . . [that] can go untreated, because there is often no-one to attend to care-giving responsibilities" (J. Hill, "The Hidden Patient," *The Lancet* 362 [2003]: 1682).

2. "Insight into why communication skills are so vital . . . picking up on unlikely verbal cues, hearing what is unsaid as much as is said, responding to body language, answering questions that are barely asked" (S. Wright, "Listen Carefully," *Nursing Standard* 18 [2004]: 27).

24

Better to Remember Him as He Was

∽

WHO SHOULD BE PART OF
THE MOURNING RITUALS?

EDNA, A WOMAN in her early seventies, knew her husband, Herman, would probably die within the week. He had been ill for about twenty months already, and the last "step down" that the disease had taken was a big one.

"I need to ask you a question."

"Ask."

"During this whole time, and I want you to know I love my children very dearly, but they have disappointed me."

"In what way?"

"Well, I wanted their help during their father's illness. But I didn't want to make them help. I wanted it to come from in here [she indicated the area of her heart]. I guess they were waiting for me to ask, but I was waiting for them to offer, and so it never came. I am very happy with them and proud of them in every other way, but I guess I expected more."

"So, Edna, what is your question?"

"Well, they have some reluctance about coming to the nursing home to see Herman. I was wondering, should I mention that maybe they would like to say goodbye? Without telling them or forcing them to, of course. Maybe it would be better for them to remember him as he was. And should they go to the funeral, or do you think it would be too much for them?"

"Edna, the easy question first. About the funeral. They are part of Herman's family, and this is a family event. You wouldn't ask them if they want to attend a family wedding. They would be expected to attend because they are part of the family. A funeral is the same. They definitely should all attend the funeral. This funeral will not be a traumatic one. This doesn't mean it won't be hard or that Herman won't be missed. However, the funeral will not be traumatic because everyone has seen this death coming for a while. It isn't a complete surprise."

"Okay. That seems right to me. It makes sense. I don't really think the funeral will present such a big problem."

"Now for the more controversial question. Should the children and grandchildren come to say goodbye to their father and grandfather? Or should they remember him as he was?"

"Edna, you have been in the front lines of Herman's care for months. From the beginning, you rightfully could have asked your children to set up a schedule of sharing the load of Herman's care with them. It is not practical to expect them to figure out that you need help with his care or visits if you are not showing this need. You don't need to 'protect' them from taking care of a man who cared for them from the time they were born till they were independent.

"They need to honor him and who he was to them regardless of whether or not he is conscious of their presence. They also need to honor you, by standing with you, in the front lines so you don't have to stand there alone. Having them there will reduce the weight of your load.

"Allowing people not to separate from their loved ones by saying either 'it may be too much for them' or 'they should remember him as he was' is another way of allowing them to abandon the dying while they are still alive. This is not acceptable. It also often causes guilt in those who remain and doesn't provide for effective closure of the relationship before the death.

"On a very practical note: after Herman dies, you are alone. If you do not expect their presence for Herman, you are giving them permission to abandon you if you become sick at some point. Do you want to 'spare' them and in the process be alone and isolated in your time of need?

"In the Ten Commandments, it says, 'Honor your father and mother that your days may be long upon the earth.' When you honor your parents with your presence and care, this enters your family repertoire and your children, who see it, are more likely to honor you in this way. Statistically, being alone can shorten your life.

"If you do not make it clear that you expect your children's and grandchildren's support, after your death your children may not receive support from their children and so on because you are allowing this to be acceptable."

We were both silent for some moments. She met my eyes waiting.

"The statement 'remember him as he was' is not accurate. Your children and grandchildren have a relationship with this man for many years. Years filled with events and memories. This weight of remembrance stands in contrast to the few minutes or hours that they are with him prior to his death. This applies even when the period is longer, as in your caring for him all these months. Compared to the decades you have had with him, this period of his illness will remain strongly in your memory for about three months and then will begin to fade, because the weight of the other memories is so much heavier.

"So, should they come to say goodbye to their father and grandfather? In a word, yes—they should all come to say goodbye. Seeing him may be difficult, but it won't be traumatic. He looks relaxed and peaceful. You can prepare them for what they will see. That means telling them ahead of time if he is connected to any machines, if he has lost weight or looks different than the last time they saw him. If he is unconscious, you want to let them know if his eyes are open or not and if his mouth is open or not."

Herman died two weeks after our conversation. Ten days later, after the formal mourning period was over, Edna met with me again. After offering condolences, we sat down with tea. Edna spoke of many things and feelings surrounding Herman's death.

"Did the children come before Herman died to say goodbye?" I asked.

"They did. It actually wasn't even my initiative that the kids came. I told them that the doctor said Herman didn't have a lot of time left. They decided to come."

"Was it good that they came?"

"They didn't tell me if it was good for them."

"What happened when they were there?"

"Well, everyone came with their spouses. Herman, as you know, was only slightly conscious and wasn't communicating at all. His eyes were closed. They spoke to him and said goodbye and that he needn't worry, they would take care of me. They said, 'Dad, we will all be all right. Good night. Sleep peacefully.' Herman suddenly had tears rolling from his eyes. They saw it was important, although it was very hard for them."

"Hard doesn't mean bad, Edna."

"Oh, I know."

"How did *you* feel?"

"I felt they were really with me. It was very good for me. The way Herman responded, we all saw it was very good for him also." She paused. "I read to him from a page in my diary where I was saying goodbye. I was looking at the page, but my children said he opened his eyes and was watching me." She sighed. "I have a lot of regrets, though. Maybe really only one regret. Although I had no choice and I had already cared for him for over a year at home, I feel badly that I had to put him in a nursing home." She looked down at her hands wrapped around her teacup and then looked up at me.

"Edna," I said quietly, "If the tables had been turned, could he have done more?"

She smiled, her eyes suddenly shining, and slowly shook her head. "No. No he couldn't."

Conclusions

- *Include many people in the support network, thereby lessening the load on each individual and also lessening the possibility of conflict or resentment between family members.*
- *All family members should attend the formal mourning rituals.*
- *Saying goodbye is not only for the benefit of the dying person but also for the one saying goodbye and for the remaining spouse.*

References

1. "Caregiving can take as little as a few hours per week, but, commonly, it is equivalent to a full-time job, with 20% of caregivers providing full-time or constant care. . . . But the sense of responsibility was never-ending. The length of a patient's illness before death and the trajectory of functional decline (and concomitant caregiving need) are difficult to predict, particularly in noncancer conditions. The administrative and logistical needs can be enormous: families typically must coordinate numerous medications, treatments, clinical and social services, as well as the needs of multiple family members. At times, families may feel as if they are 'reinventing the wheel,' with each individual family trying to identify local services even though many in their community have struggled with the very same issues. Caregivers often bear an incalculable emotional burden for their work. Although many enjoy a profound sense of privilege and derive deep satisfaction in this role, sadness, guilt, anger, resentment, and a sense of inadequacy are also common and understandable

reactions. Exhaustion, financial strain, disrupted usual activities, and continuous caregiving contribute to significant mental health morbidity, including anxiety and depression. Family caregiving can both strengthen and strain personal well-being and family relationships. Adult children frequently assume responsibilities for ill parents and may have to adjust the expectations within their own nuclear families. Amid the challenge of integrating illness into family dynamics, family members may find themselves reacquainted with long-estranged relatives during the period of end-of-life care and bereavement. Physicians can be helpful in recognizing and validating common feelings and reassuring family members about the quality of their care. Empathic responses, such as saying, 'This must be a very difficult time for you,' communicate respect and support during an emotionally stressful, even traumatic, time. In a study of 988 terminally ill patients and 893 caregivers, caregivers of patients whose physician listened to the caregivers' needs and opinions had significantly less depression (27.6%) than caregivers of similar patients with nonempathic physicians (42.0%). Adult day care, respite care, home care, social work services, and caregiver education and psychological support demonstrably improve caregiver satisfaction, quality of life, and burden. Helping family caregivers identify support resources may be especially important for families of patients ineligible for the comprehensive services provided by hospice" (M. W. Rabow, J. M. Hauser, & J. Adams, "Supporting Family Caregivers at the End of Life: 'They Don't Know What They Don't Know,'" *Journal of the American Medical Association* 291 [2004]: 483–491).

25

Waiting for Elijah

⌒

NORMAL GRIEF RESPONSES

Waiting for Elijah, he's been gone so long now
I'm waiting for Elijah, I hope he's coming soon

Here, I've gone and set a place for you, I've even filled your glass
I remember every word you said, and how they've come to pass

Even, even, eventually
And I say, even, even, eventually

And these bleeding wounds that just won't mend
and neither will the wind
White geese in the northern sky release the rainbow's end

How brightly shines the moon tonight, our words lay where they fell
Here we listen, watch and wait, I lift my ear to tell you

Even, even, eventually
And I say, even, even, eventually

Waiting for Elijah, he's been gone so long now
I'm waiting for Elijah, I hope he's coming soon

—"Waiting for Elijah"
Lyrics and music © 1970 by Peter Rowan

Michael was a high-powered security specialist in his early thirties. His only brother Marty, five years younger than Michael, had died some months earlier from a rare disease.

Michael was smart, stable, reliable, but had been badly shaken by his brother's death. He continued to function well at work, although his concentration had lost some of the edge he needed in his job. He felt he was not what he "should be" as he put it. We were meeting on a weekly basis to work through this grief.

Spring had begun, and with it the difficult period of holidays. Passover, a strong family-oriented holiday, was looming in the foreground. We discussed at some length the difficulty of such gatherings after the death of a family member.

My phone rang on the eve of Passover.

"Shalom."

"I am very sorry to disturb you on the eve of Passover."

"What is it, Michael?"

"I think I've lost my mind."

"What makes you think so?"

"This evening I'm having the whole family for the holiday meal at my home." He coughed nervously a few times.

"And?"

"And I have this irresistible urge . . ." He paused.

"What kind of urge?"

"I want to set a place at the holiday table for my brother, Marty." He was quiet again for a moment. "I know I have really lost it."

"Michael, you want to set a place for your brother, Marty, at the table? Then set a place for him at the table."

"Then it's okay? I haven't lost my mind?"

"Michael, every Passover, all around the world, every family sets a place for the prophet Elijah in case he comes back, and we don't even know him! You want to set a place for your brother? Set a place for your brother."

"But what will everyone say?"

"Everyone will say you are crazy. Tell them you spoke to your counselor about it, and she says you're not. That's all."

"Thank you so much." He breathed out in relief. "Happy Passover and I am sorry I disturbed you."

"Happy Passover to you, Michael. No problem."

Intense grief is not frequently spoken about, much like other situations surrounding the taboo subject of death. As a result, very little information about normal and abnormal responses to grief is available to the general public. This frequently makes normal responses appear frightening to the griever. How can we know whether a response is normal or not?

In this story, Michael wanted to set a place for his brother, to include him in the holiday meal through a concrete symbol. Michael didn't say, "I think my brother Marty will be at the meal." He said, "I want him to be at the meal. I want him to still be included in the family." Such symbolism is like a eulogy, a memorial. It is a way of honoring our dead. Another healthy alternative at a family event would be to raise a glass of wine also to those who "couldn't be with us here today," either by name or in a more general way.

Frequently, in an effort to return to what life was before the grief, we do the opposite of remembering and honoring our dead: we never mention the deceased family member. This is like "not talking about the elephant in the room." Everyone knows it is there but is afraid to bring the subject to the fore.

What if something really frightening happens, like the bereaved person seeing or hearing their loved one? Surprisingly, this is also normal. Seeing or hearing a deceased loved one happens to roughly a third of the grievers. Why is it important to know that this is normal? Because of our response. If we see a dead loved one while grieving and don't know it's normal, we can jump to many conclusions: "I have lost my mind," "it is a ghost," "my loved one is in trouble in the afterlife," "he is angry at me," and so on. If we know it is normal, then to see our loved ones who have died is like a shot of oxygen. It is wonderful.

What would make this grief reaction abnormal? To believe, when we see him, that he is actually back from the dead, or to insist that he hasn't died when it is clear that he has. Perhaps to hear his voice telling us what to do and feeling the need to obey it. These responses are problematic and need psychological treatment.

CONCLUSIONS

- *It is healthy to symbolically include deceased loved ones in family gatherings as a way of honoring their memory.*
- *There are different facets of grieving that may seem strange but are not abnormal.*
- *Because of the taboo nature of talking about death, the difference between normal and pathological grief responses are not widely known. This can be frightening for the griever.*

REFERENCES

1. "Grief is a painful, but unfortunately common experience. Most people at different points in their lives are confronted with the death of a close friend or relative. There are, however, marked individual differences in how intensely and how long people grieve. Some grieve openly and deeply for years, and only slowly return to a semblance of their normal level of functioning. Others suffer intensely, but for a relatively more proscribed period of time. Still others appear to get over their losses almost immediately, and to move on to new challenges and new relationships with such ease as to raise doubts among their friends and relatives as to whether they may be hiding something or running away from their pain. The extent that grief varies across individuals suggests important questions about what constitutes normal or common grief, and when, if at all, too much or too little grief might be considered abnormal, or even pathological. Unfortunately, the bereavement literature has yet to agree on a clear, empirically defensible definition of grief, or its

normal and abnormal course and manifestations" (G. A. Bonanno & S. Kaltman, "The Varieties of Grief Experience," *Clinical Psychology Review* 21 [2001]: 705–734).

2. "According to cultural anthropologists, rituals provide a standardized mode of behavior which helps to relieve the sense of uncertainty or loss. Everyone knows what to do, and how to act under those circumstances, and this restores a sense of order and continuity to their lives. It also enables the bereaved to adjust slowly to the fact of death, and to see it not as the end of one cycle, but the beginning of another. Religious and cultural rituals also comfort and reassure the mourners by helping them to make sense of death" (B. Y. Ng, "Personal Loss: Grief Revisited," *Annals of the Academy of Medicine Singapore* 34 [2005]: 352–355).

26

What Not to Say

❧

HOW TO ACT AROUND GRIEVERS

SHE RUSHED TOWARD the bathroom in tears. As she got there, the entrance was blocked by a woman going to the bathroom. Shula just pushed her into the bathroom, rushed in herself, and locked the door. She then sat down on the toilet seat and burst into bitter tears. Françoise, the woman who had initially entered the bathroom, looked on in shock.

Françoise came to Shula, squatted down near her, and put her hand on her knee in silence. Shula continued to cry for several long minutes. Looking up, she took the proffered toilet paper from Françoise's hand, wiped her face, and stood up. "Thanks. I'm sorry. Could you leave for a moment so I can use the bathroom?" Françoise silently nodded and left the bathroom, her own bladder nearly bursting.

A few moments later they traded places, and Shula went back to the mourners who had gathered to comfort her family after the death of her son. A woman came to her and said emphatically,

"Shula, if it was me ... if it had been my son, I would die! How can you stand it?" Shula looked at her in horror, realizing the implications. *What, I am supposed to die now? Is that what this woman expects? How could she say such a callous thing?* Shula's daughter, Tali, interrupted and said to her mother, "Mom, you have a phone call. I'll go with you." Shula looked at her gratefully and pried herself away from the "comforter."

The past three days since Yosi's death had been a nightmare. And on top of all of the shock and horror, there were these "comforters," well-meaning friends, coworkers, and neighbors, always saying the wrong thing. She remembered a litany of comments that she had heard here:

"Be strong." Excellent advice, but how and why be strong now when it was time to cry?

"Everything will be okay"? What on earth, what exactly was going to be okay now that her son was dead?

Or the famous "Time heals all things." What do they know? Have they lost a brother, a son?

There were those who said, "May you know no more sorrow." A nice sentiment, Shula mused, but three days after her son's death, and eight months after her father's fatal heart attack, she felt the only way to "know no more sorrow" was by dying herself. The people who came, who Shula had never seen before and who never even met Yosi and yet they had the nerve to say, "I share your sorrow." Really!

Then there were the comforters who didn't say anything about Yosi but instead wanted to tell Shula all about the deaths they had had to go through, in painstaking detail. Like there wasn't enough death in this house already.

Shula's thoughts were interrupted when she heard a man, who had cornered her husband Joshua nearby, saying, "Yosi died for nothing, for nothing at all! Such a waste." How could he say that to Yosi's father! She saw Joshua's fists clenching and unclenching as he tried to control his emotions.

Meanwhile, Tali, still standing with her mother, was met by yet another "comforter"—this one bearing sage advice: "Now you are the oldest child, Tali. You must take over all the things your brother did. You need to take care of your parents."

Shula quickly turned to her daughter and said, "Tali, you are *not* the oldest. Yosi will always be the oldest, whether or not he is alive. And you are not to take care of me. I am the mother and I will take care of you. I know this woman means well, but she is mistaken."

Probably the worst for Shula was the response of some of her close friends. Not all of them, mind you, only those who tried to change the subject every time she brought up Yosi's name. She even asked Karen, after the third time she had done this, "Why did you come here?"

Karen replied, "To comfort you."

"Then why won't you let me talk about Yosi?"

"Because I see how much it hurts you, and I want to protect you," Karen replied sheepishly.

"Just let me talk and cry, okay? I really need to."

What is wrong or inappropriate about all of the things mentioned above that Shula heard?

Mourners are in a very vulnerable state following the death of their loved one. Things said lightly or thoughtlessly can be taken very hard, as any counselor has certainly heard from grievers, or any mourner has experienced in their own time of grief.

What should we say when we want to help a griever? There are two parts to the answer. The first part is: why do we feel we need to say something when there is nothing to say?

What we actually say as we enter a house of mourning usually has no communication value. It has rather a ceremonial value. The real message is: "I am here. I have come to see you or comfort you, in your grief."

One appropriate way to enter a house of mourning is silently. Approach the griever that you have come to comfort, put a hand on his shoulder, or shake his hand. Sometimes people bring food to share or flowers; depending on the culture, this may also be appropriate.

We often feel compelled to speak "comforting words" rather than remain silent due to our own discomfort, bewilderment, and helplessness. We offer unwanted or erroneous advice to try to be "helpful" to the grievers. We steer mourners away from dwelling on their loss because we find that witnessing their pain is hard for us to bear.

So what would be appropriate to say? If we want to help the person who is mourning, the best way is to invite them to speak through an open question. Perhaps, "How did you find out?" Or in cases where the deceased is not known to the comforter, "I never really knew him. Could you tell me about him?" Sometimes, it is appropriate to share a good memory of the deceased that his family may not know about. This is giving them a gift to hold on to. "How are you holding up?" is another appropriate question. If the mourner doesn't want to speak, sit with them in silence. This is frequently a greater comfort than words.

> ## Conclusions
>
> - *It is difficult to go into a house of mourning. You don't have to have all of the right words. Frequently silence is a more helpful option.*
> - *It is most helpful for mourners to speak about their grief. Open questions are the best way to facilitate this.*

References

1. "The physician's discomfort or uncertainty about what to say or do when encountering a bereaved patient must be overcome in favor of taking active steps to help them. A list of comments and practices in communicating with and caring for grieving patients has been derived from a synthesis of discussions with widowed persons, participation in grief support groups, and suggestions offered by various Web sites. Putting upsetting experiences into words, including disclosure about emotions in response to the death of a spouse, is associated with improved physical and mental health. Written and oral disclosure studies have even demonstrated a positive influence on immune function. Based on these findings, physicians might encourage bereaved patients to express their thoughts and feelings about the loss (e.g., in a journal)" (H. G. Prigerson & S. C. Jacobs, "Caring for Bereaved Patients: 'All the Doctors Just Suddenly Go,'" *Journal of the American Medical Association* 286 [2001]: 1369–1376).

What Is Yours, What Is Not

∾

Empathy, Boundaries, Identification

"I HAVE DIAGNOSED and accompanied from diagnosis to death dozens of children . . . perhaps over a hundred," he said with great emotion. "Each child was like my own child." Tears were filling his eyes.

Everyone in the staff meeting was affected. As he spoke, I could hear sniffling and see people wiping away tears with sleeves or tissue.

The speaker was Jacob, a physician who treated children with infectious diseases. He and his staff were interviewing me to do staff support in this difficult unit.

He continued, "Frequently, the bereaved parents even comfort me. They see how greatly I loved their child." I looked around and saw that everyone in the room was in tears, including Jacob. Everyone except me. Inwardly churning, I waited. Jacob turned to me. He waited for my response. It was not long in coming.

Leaning toward him, I said quietly, "The only reason you can say that each of these children was like your own child is because *none* of them *was* your own child."

After a pause, I continued. "You go home to your healthy children, and you say you are bereaved like a parent who returns to the empty house, the empty bed, the empty chair at the table? They see the friends and siblings of their child grow older, feeling all the pain of no future, where so much future was planned." I waited for the words to sink in. Shock registered on all of their faces.

"This reaction of yours is unacceptable, unethical, unprofessional, and if I accept your proposition to train your staff, it will not happen here again."

Surprisingly, at the close of this interview, I was given the job.

It is not an uncommon problem in the helping professions to blur the boundaries between "what is mine" and "what is yours." One important way to prevent this is by recognizing the difference between your own pain and someone else's pain.

Let's start with what is yours: people who are important to you and/or who were important to you prior to the trauma or tragedy are yours, and the loss of them is also your loss. These are frequently people with whom you share a common history. People whose absence hurts you personally, in the course of your life, not only at work, are yours. Their absence may change your daily schedule or leave tasks and roles empty that were once filled by the deceased.

What is not yours? Loss that hurts someone you care about. Helplessness at being unable to turn the tide of illness, injury, or death of someone you know or are caring for in a professional capacity. This is someone else's loss. It's not *your* loss.

Sometimes it is difficult to identify what belongs to whom because you can sense someone else's pain so strongly. That is their pain. That pain is not yours.

In the main, people who choose to work with dying children—nurses, physicians, and psychosocial workers—are exceptional people. But these same people frequently burn out under the emotional stress of their work. It is important to make the differentiation between what is yours and what is not because if you are personally involved, your ability to help is more limited. This is contrary to popular belief. You are more limited because if you take the grief personally, then you also have to take care of yourself. You have less remaining energy for the other person. Your view is distorted, that is, seen through the lens of your own grief.

The recognition of what is "not mine" allows professionals an adequate emotional distance to function as support for the long term. This is another reason that it is easier to help a stranger than someone who knows you. Because they don't know you, they don't need to be distracted by your personhood; they can just be "on the stage" and speak about their own experience. This empathy (see reference 1 below) allows the other person, with his pain, to feel understood, respected, and validated. This person is allowed to have his "own" pain. His loss is recognized as his own personal experience, and he is accorded the right to express it as he sees fit, without having to compete for the stage with others who "also suffer" with him.

Some of the ways to help the bereaved feel understood and respected involve active listening. Active listening uses both words and body language:

> MAKE EYE CONTACT. Don't try to do anything else (like writing or looking at a computer screen or paper) while you are listening.

> MAKE SURE YOU understand what is being said. For this, it is useful to use phrases such as "Let's see if I have this right..." or "You are saying...?" and then repeat what they told you in different words. If you don't get confirmation, you aren't finished.

> IDENTIFY AND CALIBRATE the emotion you feel from them: "I have the feeling that you feel strongly about this; can you be more specific?"

> REQUEST AND ACCEPT CORRECTION: "Did I leave anything out?"

CONCLUSIONS

- *In order to effectively help another person, it is important to know what is yours and what is not.*
- *In order to protect yourself from burnout, you also need to know what is yours and what is not.*
- *Active listening is important when dealing with grief.*

REFERENCES

1. "In clinical medicine, empathy is the ability to understand the patient's situation, perspective and feelings and to communicate that understanding to the patient. The effective use of empathy promotes diagnostic accuracy, therapeutic adherence and patient satisfaction, while remaining time-efficient. Empathy also enhances physician satisfaction. As with any other tool, clinical empathy requires systematic practice to achieve mastery" (J. L. Coulehan, F. W. Platt, B. Egener, R. Frankel, C. T. Lin, B. Lown, & W. H. Salazar, " 'Let Me See If I Have This Right . . .': Words That Help Build Empathy," *Annals of Internal Medicine* 135 [2001]: 221–227).

2. "Doctors still often feel that a patient's death is a personal failure, which can cause the physician to withdraw. Caring physicians have been said to exhibit two primary attributes— receptivity and responsibility—which they translate into excellent clinical practice. Some exude a professional 'detached concern.' Whatever the style, *active listening* is therapy for the patient, while, for the clinician, it is a remarkable opportunity to learn how people make sense of their lives and the crisis of approaching death" (R. T. Penson, R. A. Partridge, M. A. Shah, D. Giansiracusa, B. A. Chabner, & T. J. Lynch Jr., "Fear of Death," *Oncologist* 10, no. 2 [2005]: 160–169).

28

Laugh and the World Laughs . . .

∽

WHEN YOU ARE DYING,
YOU ARE STILL ALIVE

The secret source of humor itself is not joy but sorrow.
　　　　　　　　—Mark Twain, *Following the Equator*

SIXTY-FOUR-YEAR-OLD EYAL had been diagnosed with cancer of the liver—"in the middle of life," he mourned. The bad news had come eight months ago, and Eyal was angry all the time. We had been meeting for about three weeks.

　　Eyal turned to me and said, "I have written a poem. It was even published this week in the newspaper. Would you like to see it?"

　　"Yes."

　　He showed me his poem:

10 Things I Have to Do Today:

Inhale

Exhale

Inhale

Exhale

Inhale

Exhale

Inhale

Exhale

Inhale

Exhale

I burst out laughing. Eyal looked shocked. He began to smile. "No one else laughed when I showed it to them. Why did you laugh?"

"Because it's funny."

He perused the poem again with a smile, and then he began to laugh a bit also. We both laughed louder and louder. He had tears of laughter streaming from his eyes.

He breathed in deeply to calm down.

"Why is it so funny?" he asked.

"Probably because it's so true."

He smiled, and our meeting continued.

Now, in a different tone, he began to tell me of all the confusing and slapstick moments in the hospital. A lot of this time was spent in black humor, laughing at things that had angered and frustrated him at the time.

When the meeting was over, he went out to the garden. His wife, Miriam, came from another room in the house for our meeting.

"What was going on in here!?" she asked.

"What do you mean?"

"Since Eyal was diagnosed eight months ago, there has been no laughter in this house. Now we have a grief counselor here, and I hear almost an hour of continuous laughter. What were you talking about?"

"About death, sickness, frustration, and anger. Some sadness and helplessness too."

"Then why were you laughing so much?"

"Laughter is the emotion closest to crying, but it doesn't have the stigma of lack of control or being feminine. It is a release valve for tension, anger, and grief."

Dying people are still alive. And as such, the whole repertoire of human emotions is open to them. The problem is, we don't know how to approach someone who is dying, so we do it on tiptoes, with great gravity, sadness, and fear. This effectively limits the dying person's acceptable range of responses.

CONCLUSIONS

- *Dying people are still alive and deserve to be treated as such. This includes allowing them to respond with all of the emotions they have.*
- *Laughter is many times close to tears and, like tears, is an effective release valve for emotion.*

REFERENCES

1. Laughter, and the broader category of humor, are key elements in helping us go on with our life after a loss. Laughter lifts us up. Humor can alter any situation and help us cope at the very instant we are laughing. Humor allows us to cope with both physical and mental pain in three ways: (1) When we are dealing with death we are constantly being dragged down by the event; humor diverts our attention and lifts our sagging spirits. (2) Dealing with death is stressful; humor decreases our stress and tension. (3) In the midst of death, life feels out of balance; humor provides that balance by providing a fresh perspective and power in a powerless situation. . . . When we are in pain and wish that something would 'take us away from all of this' humor does exactly that. It may be for only a brief moment but it distracts us from our pain and gives us hope to embrace life again. If we can laugh again, we can live again" (A. Klein, "Laughter and Loss," www.allenklein.com/articles/laughterandloss.htm, accessed January 12, 2007).

2. According to Bill Cosby, "if you can find humor in anything . . . you can survive it."

3. "Although researchers in a number of disciplines have studied the effects of humor on patients, limited work has focused on end-of-life care. The present study. . . . Results revealed that

humor was present in 85 percent of 132 observed nurse-based hospice visits. . . . hospice patients initiated humor 70 percent of the time. . . . Humor was spontaneous and frequent, and instances of humorous interactions were a prevalent part of everyday hospice work" (K. N. Adamle & R. Ludwick, "Humor in Hospice Care: Who, Where, and How Much?" *American Journal of Hospice and Palliative Care* 22 [2005]: 287–290).

4. "Clients and team members used humor to build relationships, contend with circumstances, and express sensibilities. . . . Participants relied on intuition as well as a constellation of other factors in discerning whether or not to use humor. Techniques for assessment included identification of cues such as expression in the eyes and timing as indications of receptivity. Combined with caring and sensitivity, humor is a powerful therapeutic asset in hospice/palliative care. It must neither be taken for granted nor considered trivial" (R. A. Dean & D. M. Gregory, "More Than Trivial: Strategies for Using Humor in Palliative Care," *Cancer Nurs*ing 28 [2005]: 292–300).

29

The Minefield

~

NORMAL GRIEF

I MET WITH JOANNE again this week. She looked like a wreck. She was chain smoking.

"What's up?"

"You didn't warn me."

"Excuse me?"

"You didn't warn me about the minefield from yesterday."

"What minefield is that?"

"I stood by my window, crying, sobbing, as I watched all the other kids in the neighborhood. They were all dressed up in new clothes. All with new backpacks. And I knew exactly what was in their backpacks. New pencil cases, sharpened pencils and crayons, some paper, a few markers, scissors and maybe a stapler. Some white glue . . . and a lunch in a small bag, made with love." Joanne's voice had been rising and ended with a muffled cry. She began to sob and rock herself back and forth in front of the window.

She wiped her nose with Kleenex and began again. "Sorry." She inhaled her cigarette deeply and sighed it out, staring out at the street. "I was standing right here. I can still see them all. But not my Randy. It will never be my Randy out there with them again."

At the moment we learn of the death of a loved one, we enter an emotional "minefield." Each "mine" is a flood of feelings, either expressed or unexpressed, depending on personality and cultural expectations.

Many of the "mines" are unexpected, but some of them we can prepare for, for example: the deceased's birthday for the first time since his death, our birthday without the loved one, family holidays, weekends, or other blocks of time we used to spend with the loved one. There are also other "mines" that can surface without advance warning: songs on the radio that remind us of our loved ones, unofficial anniversaries, a whiff of their favorite perfume, food smells that bring back memories, mail arriving for them after their death, people meeting us and offering condolences in public places without warning, or phone calls from those who didn't know they had died. Other triggers might be places they loved, hated, or that are associated somehow with their death, hearing their name when it refers to someone else, and more.

As in the above story, a predictable minefield is the first day of school for parents bereaved of small children.

How big is this minefield? How long will it last?

Most of the mines will have been stepped on or triggered by the time the first anniversary arrives (one year after the death). There are also "mines" that can come after the first year: weddings, births, deaths where the deceased's absence is felt. But, by the end of the first year, we know where most of the mines are, and we have an idea on how we personally can best cope with them.

How can we prepare for the mines? Knowing that they are coming is one way. We can steel ourselves somewhat for the encounters. Sometimes it is best not to plan any unnecessary activities for the days that we know will be harder. In some cases, we can choose whether to be in public or not.

CONCLUSIONS

- *Following the death of a significant person, we can expect floods of feelings to be triggered by many events.*
- *Some "mines" are predictable, but many are not.*
- *We can lessen, somewhat, the emotional stress by preparing for known triggers and by knowing that there will be surprise mines now and then.*

REFERENCES

1. " 'Pangs of grief'—the intrusive, time-limited intense yearning and pining for the deceased—may come and go in waves for years after the loss" (H. G. Prigerson & S. C. Jacobs, "Caring for Bereaved Patients: 'All the Doctors Just Suddenly Go,' " *Journal of the American Medical Association* 286 [2001]: 1369–1376).

2. "Grief is not a steady process. Grief spasms, described by Rando as an 'upsurge of grief that occurs suddenly and often when least expected,' can occur at any time. The emotional reactions in a grief spasm can be very intense, although temporary. While these spasms of grief are normal, they can be triggered by

nothing in particular or by something that usually elicits little reaction, such as a visit to the physician, especially if the physician also cared for the deceased. Triggers can occur long after the bereaved have resolved much of their grief" (N. A. Carrington & J. F. Bogetz, "Normal Grief and Bereavement: Letters from Home," *Journal of Palliative Medicine* 7 [2004]: 309–323).

30

I Want to Finish His Life for Him

∽

IDENTIFICATION OF BEREAVED SIBLINGS WITH THE DECEASED

THE LIVING ROOM and dining room were filled to overflowing with people who came to offer their condolences. There must have been over seventy people in the small rooms. They stood or sat in groups, talking quietly. Sighs and occasional sniffles could be heard throughout. There were identifiable groups among them: friends and classmates, many soldiers, among them those who were with Abraham in his last battle at the Lebanon front. Family was sitting, slumped or cradling their heads heavily in their hands, pained or dull looks on their faces. Two of Abraham's younger siblings were moving slowly around the room, marking their parents with concern. The third sat in a chair, surrounded by friends, silent at the young age of six, tissue clutched in her fist.

The oldest of the siblings, Dawn, age nine, came to her mother and placed her hand on her head. "Mom?"

"Yes, honey."

"Mom, what did Abraham want to be when he grows up?" she asked.

"I don't know, sweetheart," her mother said quietly. "He thought about many things," she paused and sighed heavily. "Maybe a doctor, or a computer programmer, perhaps a photographer." She met Dawn's eyes again. "Why do you ask?"

"Because I want to finish his life for him," Dawn answered seriously.

Dawn's mother's eyes widened in alarm with the memory of other soldiers who had died, trying to finish the lives of their fathers or brothers who had died before them in the army.

Susanna, a close friend of the family, had been following the interchange. She smiled sadly. "Oh, Dawn, that is wonderful. You are such a good girl."

Dawn's mother reached out suddenly filled with fear and took Dawn by the upper arms. She drew her closer while looking seriously into her eyes. "Dawn, beloved, no, you cannot finish Abraham's life for him, because Abraham's life is over." She tightened her lips with determination and continued. "Dawn, if you want to be an author and write a book that you dedicate to Abraham, you can do that." She paused, searching Dawn's face, and continued. "If you want to be a scientist and discover something and name it for Abraham, you can do that. If you want to be a singer and sing a song written for Abraham, you can do that too." She took a deep breath. "But you cannot be Abraham, any more than Abraham could ever have been you. You need to be the best Dawn that you can be, and no one else." She hugged Dawn so tightly, squeezing her eyes tight against the horrific thought of losing yet another child.

Bereaved siblings are most at risk for identifying strongly with the deceased sibling even to the point of wanting to become the deceased child. Why?

When a family is bereaved of a child, the remaining children see their parents in a situation that they have probably never seen before. It may be one of the rare times they have seen one or both of their parents cry or cease to function. The deceased child not only becomes the center of attention, but the parents, neutralized by grief, have no attention for the remaining children.

The remaining children see how strongly the parents grieve over the lost sibling and how their parents have no energy left for them. They begin to feel that "it probably would have been easier for my parents had I died and my sibling lived." In order to comfort the parents, and/or to find a place again in their parents' lives, the sibling tries to "replace" the deceased sibling, to become as much like him as possible. This may take the form of changing a direction of interest from their own to that of the deceased sibling or moving to the deceased child's room or bed. With older siblings, it may mean dating the former girl/boyfriend of the deceased, wearing the deceased sibling's clothing exclusively, taking up the mannerisms of the deceased, and so on.

Family members or comforters who come to the home or place of mourning following the death might mistakenly encourage this, or even suggest to the sibling closest in age, or the sibling of the same sex as the deceased, to become a replacement with statements like "Now you are the oldest," or "It is so wonderful that you want to carry on your sibling's life for him." This is further sanctioned by the fact that we tend to idealize the dead, thereby making the deceased sibling into someone perfect, not resembling a normal human being.

We cannot, by sheer willpower, become someone else. However, we can choose to abandon, by an act of will, who *we* are. The result is that we will "fall between the chairs" so to speak, and develop into neither one nor the other, without a fully rounded personality.

It is very important to validate the surviving siblings' right to continue to live their own lives rather than replace the lives of the deceased. Other ways can be found to honor lost loved ones.

CONCLUSIONS

- *Bereaved siblings sometimes feel obligated to replace the deceased sibling.*
- *Despite the fact that family and well-meaning observers sometimes applaud this as a fitting tribute to the deceased, it is problematic for the sibling.*
- *It is important to give explicit permission and direction to remaining children to continue to be who they are and not try to replace their deceased sibling.*

REFERENCES

1. "No one ever told me that grief felt so like fear" (C. S. Lewis, *A Grief Observed* [London: Faber and Faber, 1961], p. 7.

2. "As parents remember the baby who has died, care should be taken not to idealize this baby or indicate in any way that the subsequent children can replace the deceased child or that the subsequent child is not as good as the child that died" (Anonymous, "Helping Subsequent Children Learn about Their SIDS Siblings" *Silver Lining Newsletter* 1, no. 1 [spring 2006]: 7). at

http://www.sidsillinois.org/images/reading_material/newsspring
2006.pdf accessed February 9, 2007).

3. "When a child is born into a family that has suffered a loss, there is concern that the new child might be compromised in his or her development. Such a baby is often described as a 're-placement child,' a substitute or replacement for the child who died. This baby is thought to be at risk for later psychological difficulties because of an inability to form an identity separate from the dead child. It is thought that parents who are unable to fully and completely mourn the death of their child may com-promise a subsequent child's mental health by imbuing that child with the qualities and characteristics of the dead sibling and by continuing to mourn the earlier death" (Replacement Children forum, Encyclopedia of Death and Dying, www .deathreference.com/Py-Se/Replacement-Children.html, ac-cessed February 10, 2007).

4. "Parents' thinking about the dead baby and about the new baby may result in problematic parent-child relationships by creating an environment in which the new baby functions to replace the dead child. . . . This phenomenon is known in the clinical arena as the 'replacement child,' and may be one way in which parents represent their families in the long term after a loss. . . . It seems already clear, however, that clinical axioms like 'replacement child' do not do justice to the complexity of parental representations of the child and the family constella-tion. Without understanding the constructed meanings of the dead child and subsequent children, without listening closely to the stories parents tell, clinicians are in danger of assuming risk when there may be none" (L. A. Grout & B. D. Romanoff, "The Myth of the Replacement Child: Parents' Stories and Practices after Perinatal Death," *Death Studies* 24[2000]: 93).